OF FOXES
AND HEN HOUSES

New Titles from QUORUM BOOKS

The Export-Import Bank at Work: Promotional Financing in the
Public Sector
JORDAN JAY HILLMAN

Supply-Side Economics in the 1980s: Conference Proceedings
FEDERAL RESERVE BANK OF ATLANTA AND EMORY UNIVERSITY LAW AND
ECONOMICS CENTER, SPONSORS

Deregulation and Environmental Quality: The Use of Tax Policy to
Control Pollution in North America and Western Europe
CRAIG E. REESE

Danger: Marketing Researcher at Work
TERRY HALLER

OPEC, the Petroleum Industry, and United States Energy Policy
ARABINDA GHOSH

Corporate Internal Affairs: A Corporate and Securities Law Perspective
MARC I. STEINBERG

International Pharmaceutical Marketing
SURESH B. PRADHAN

Social Costs in Modern Society: A Qualitative and Quantitative
Assessment
JOHN E. ULLMANN, EDITOR

Animal Law
DAVID S. FAVRE AND MURRAY LORING

Competing for Capital in the '80s: An Investor Relations Approach
BRUCE W. MARCUS

The International Law of Pollution: Protecting the Global Environment in a
World of Sovereign States
ALLEN L. SPRINGER

Statistical Concepts for Attorneys: A Reference Guide
WAYNE C. CURTIS

Handbook of Record Storage and Spacement Management
C. PETER WAEGEMANN

Industrial Bonds and the Rating Process
AHMED BELKAOUI

OF FOXES AND HEN HOUSES

Licensing and the Health Professions

STANLEY J. GROSS

Q QUORUM BOOKS

WESTPORT, CONNECTICUT
LONDON, ENGLAND

Library of Congress Cataloging in Publication Data

Gross, Stanley J.
  Of foxes and hen houses.

  Bibliography: p.
  Includes index.
  1. Medical personnel—Licenses—United States.
I. Title. [DNLM: 1. Licensure—United States. 2. Health
occupations—United States. W 40 AA1 G80]
RA396.A3G73 1984   610'.7   83-11218
ISBN 0-89930-059-6 (lib. bdg.)

Library of Congress Catalog Card Number: 83-11218
ISBN: 0-89930-059-6

First published in 1984 by Quorum Books

Greenwood Press
A division of Congressional Information Service, Inc.
88 Post Road West, Westport, Connecticut 06881

Printed in the United States of America

10 9 8 7 6 5 4 3 2 1

Acknowledgments

Some portions of this book were revised from the following articles and chapter:

Professional Disclosure: An Alternative to Licensure, *Personnel and Guidance Journal*, 1977,
55(10) 568-588. Copyright (1977) American Personnel and Guidance Association. Reprinted
with permission. No further reproduction authorized without written permission of APGA.

The Myth of Professional Licensing, *American Psychologist*, 1978, *33*(11) 1009-1016.
Copyright (1978) by the American Psychological Association. Reprinted by permission of the
publisher.

Public Policy Implications for Studies on Licensing and Competency. *The Rutgers Professional
Psychology Review*, 1980, 2:5-14. Copyright (1980) Graduate School of Applied and
Professional Psychology, Rutgers, The State University of New Jersey. Reprinted with
permission.

Holistic Perspective on Professional Licensing, *Journal of Holistic Medicine*, 1981, 3(1) 38-45.
Copyright (1981) Human Sciences Press. Reprinted with permission.

The Professional as Regulator and Self-Regulator from *Power and Conflict in Continuing
Professional Education* by Milton R. Stern, editor. Copyright (1983) by Wadsworth, Inc.
Reprinted by permission of Wadsworth Publishing Company. Belmont, California 94002.

The author and publisher also wish to acknowledge permission to reprint material from:
E. Freidson, *Professional dominance*, New York, Aldine, 1970, pp. 4, 66, 68, 70, 83, 197, 215,
219, 226, 235; R. Collins, *The credential society: An historical sociology of education and
stratification*, New York, Academic Press, 1979, pp. 13, 79, 134, 135, 173, 178, 198; and J. K.
Lieberman, *The tyranny of the experts*, New York, Walker & Co., 1970, pp. 57, 108-9, 137,
246, 282.

To my parents,
Selma Krebs Gross and
Albert S. Gross

CONTENTS

TABLES

PREFACE

The image of a fox guarding a hen house depicts the situation of professionals charged with regulating themselves to protect the public. As a consequence of self-regulation they have been able to ignore the substantial amount of evidence that has rejected the assumption that self-regulation has safeguarded the public. It is the purpose of this book to synthesize this evidence and bring it to the attention of the public and its policymakers.

This book is an interdisciplinary examination of one form of self-regulation—professional licensure—and the problem it poses for public policy. Licensing has failed to ensure competency and honesty in professional service and instead has given special status to professionals at a heavy social and economic cost. The monopoly and autonomy granted by licensure support professional standards that disregard the public interest and encourage relationships with clients based on mystification and dependency so that the public supports the very system that exploits and harms them.

My interest in professional licensure as a topic for study was stimulated by chance. I had read and heard proposals in the mid-1970s that counselors, social workers, and other health and helping professionals should pursue licensing to protect their occupational turf against encroachment by restrictive licensing acts being passed for other professions (for example, psychology). Though I was distressed by this turn of events, I felt stymied by the lack of an alternative to licensing. In the spring of 1976, however, I attended the Midwest Conference of the Association for Humanistic Psychology, where I happened onto an informal meeting called by Diane Reifler, then training director at the OASIS Center for Human Potential. Diane talked about a successful attempt to defeat a counselor licensing bill in the Illinois legislature. She referred to something she called a professional disclosure statute, which she suggested as an alternative to licensure. The idea that accurate information could offer greater protection than the "presumption of competence" offered by licensure was an eye-opener to me at the time.

Investigating professional disclosure, I made a discovery that confirmed my uneasiness about licensure and that would sustain and direct my research and writing for the next five years—the library shelves were full of research and scholarly analyses, which almost without exception were highly critical of licensing. After I listened to and read the discussions of licensing by professionals and consumers, it was also apparent that this abundant literature was being ignored. My own attempts to bring the research into discussions with professional colleagues earned the type of pat on the head some reserve for an eager but naive student who does not understand the politics of a situation.

Even scholarly work in licensing reflects the type of myopia pictured by blind men examining an elephant. With a few exceptions (Hogan, 1979a), scholars in the separate disciplines ordinarily do not build on each other's work. A comprehensive examination of licensure has not been available and this book attempts to bridge the gap. Making use of the separate insights of economists, sociologists, psychologists, historians, political scientists, and lawyers has been an interdisciplinary adventure for me. There was so much material available that, in a sense, the book seemed to write itself. That it could be written using the resources of a comparatively small university library and its excellent interlibrary loan staff is testimony to the wealth of material available. This is an issue so rich in scholarship and so well ignored that I felt a strong urge to write about it. At the same time, I have been concerned about being true to the material and not sensationalizing it. It has been a challenge to understand the perspectives of the separate disciplines, and I hope I have done them justice.

I began with a concern about licensing in counseling and psychology, but it soon became apparent that the problem had to do with the dynamics of professionalism generally. The impact of technology on the health professions, the competition for third-party payments, and the fascination by sociologists with the medical profession, all provided a wealth of material about the health professions particularly and suggested a more restricted focus. It is appropriate that medicine be singled out for special attention. Medicine is the subject of much research and scholarship, and it is the model to which other professions aspire. Experience with that model is instructive since the scenario of medical licensing has been repeated by other health professions as well as nonhealth professions. Consequently, the ultimate target for these comments is the licensing system operated by the states for all professions and occupations.

The title *Of Foxes and Hen Houses* suggests a perspective. The bulk of research and scholarship is clearly critical of licensing. I have taken it to mean that it is not just the current licensing system that is faulty, but that licensure is inherently defective. Licensure needs to be replaced by systems that enhance self-protection and choice. The licensing system appears to be highly resistant to change because of the entrenched power of professionals and the mystification of the public, but it is vulnerable. It rests on the notion that it protects the public. Protection is the basis for the use of the states' constitutionally derived police powers to restrict freedom of choice of an occupation or of a practitioner. Professional licensure is a house of cards that may be tumbled by the wind of consumer information and awareness.

Though reference is made throughout the book to professional self-interest and to lack of accountability, no implication should be drawn that individual practitioners or professional associations are intentionally self-serving. In fact, an important reason for the book is that professionals, too, are taken in by the myth of protecting the public, but they do not distinguish between what is good for them and what is good for the public, nor do they demonstrate the will to solve the myriad problems posed by licensure. There may not be a deliberate attempt to delude the public, but the effect is the same. Professionals benefit unreasonably from licensure through enhanced earnings, prestige, and career security. This has raised questions about the credibility of professionals and may very well jeopardize the special prerogatives and privileges accorded to them.

The reader I have in mind is a person who may have read in the newspapers about the recent attempt by the American Medical Association to gain an exemption from Federal Trade Commission investigations of anticompetitive business practices; he is a legislator being asked to support still another health association's bid for licensing legislation; she is a licensing board member concerned about criticism of board functioning; he, while studying to become a health professional, wonders why credentials that may be satisfactory in Illinois are not in California; she cannot understand the common prohibition against home birthing by midwives; he wonders about the disciplinary activities of many health professions' licensing boards. These people also ask, *what is this business of licensing about?* My intention is to bring together information about licensing so as to forge an understanding of the phenomenon in the minds of persons who would choose to do something to change it. I have the hope that the action would lead to an increase in freedom of choice and self-protection.

Despite the fact that I have been trained in counseling and psychology and not as a sociologist or a social psychologist, I have read in these disciplines for many years. This reading influenced and prepared me to undertake this project by making a social structure perspective available to me. The way we look at phenomena is critical in determining what we see, whether we act, and, if so, how we act on such information. One way of viewing phenomena is not necessarily better than other ways, it is merely different. Judgments of better or worse are determined by the goals we seek and the actions we take to achieve them. When a social structure perspective is used, we change the focus of our lens from the harder, sharper focus on the content of the happenings and experiences of individuals in the social setting to the softer, more diffuse focus on the beliefs and values people bring to situations and the implicit rules and expectations affecting the contexts within which they act. Thus, in the case of professional licensure, we are more interested in describing the social supports for monopoly and autonomy than the specifics, for example, of the legislation that actually grants these privileges.

Improving the quality of professional service requires attention to the social structure of the relationship between the professional and the client. Problems that limit quality are seen, in the perspective developed here, to derive from the social and economic incentives that affect how clients and health professionals relate to one another rather than from the professional's personality or training. These incentives produce the accepted standards of professions that, in turn, affect the behavior of health professionals and that are known to frustrate peer review, block client feedback, encourage client dependence, and support impersonal behavior.

Freidson (1970), referring to the medical profession, concludes that "the present organization of medical practice systematically encourages the *average* physician to give indifferent medical care" (p. 70). This way of looking at the problem follows an approach labeled "structuralist" that centers on the power of social institutions and processes to shape individual behavior. Freidson takes the position that the social environment reinforces behavior, thus, it may "lead people to forsake one set of motives, values, or knowledge in favor of another" (p. 66). This means wherever we observe behavior in a population that is internally consistent, ordered, and almost universally similar, as we find with regard to professional licensure, we should also find, in Alford's (1975) term, a "dominant structural interest" in the sociocultural environment. Alford, in fact, points to professional monopoly as an example of a dominant structural interest, whereby "existing institutions protect and reinforce the logic and principle of professional monopoly over the production and distribution of health services" (p. 14). Professional monopolists need not continuously organize and act to defend their interests; they have it done for them. The dominant structural interest, in effect, creates a self-fulfilling prophecy for certain socially valued behaviors. Its pervasiveness and invisibility make it extremely resistant to planned change strategies.

Freidson (1970) uses a clear, if unlikely, example to show what happens if we ignore social structure and emphasize only what individuals can do.

Imagine building housing without fire escapes, fire retardant materials, or sprinkler systems. Instead, reliance is put on educating the public to be careful with matches and small boys and on teaching them where plastic surgeons can be found when small boys succeed and first aid fails. Public figures deplore the shortage of plastic surgeons and the Burn Foundation has a March of Dollars so as to be able to pour resources into improving clinical knowledge about burns and into caring for the indigent burned. Social policy focuses on "educating" prospective patients and grinding out enough physicians or physician-substitutes in order to serve the large number of patients who were not successfully educated. [p. 68]

Change in the direction of protecting the public, if it is to be meaningful rather than cosmetic, thus necessitates alterations in our social, political, and economic institutions so that different dominant structural interests are encouraged. The thesis will be developed that, since licensing is at the crux of a credentialing system which is monopolistic and autonomous, changes in licensing regulations that enhance competition and accountability will create other changes which will shape professional service to raise quality, reduce cost, and increase public self-protection.

Also fundamental to the approach here is Freidson's idea (Bloom and Wilson, 1972) that the current licensing arrangements are the result of bargaining between the interests of two distinct social systems in client-professional relationships. According to Freidson, it is not just the professional who is responsible for the dominant-submissive relationship; the system meets the needs of the client, too. Ehrenreich (1978) recognized this circumstance observing that "the dependency and passivity characteristic of modern medical care are sought by patients as well as imposed by doctors; they reflect not only the interests of the doctors and of giant corporations, but also the needs of patients." (p. 22). This explains the public's resistance to changing the system even though that system doesn't appear to function in the public interest. The public has tolerated dependency because gaining access to the information necessary for self-determination is difficult and also because the possibility of being abandoned by professionals is threatening. The payoff for the public is that experts are seen to order an otherwise chaotic and dangerous world. Any effective approach to the problems licensing poses must grasp the twin realities of social structure and bargaining among distinct social systems.

It would not have been possible to complete this book without the aid of many people, most of whom were associated with Indiana State University. A sabbatical leave in the spring semester of 1980 and later adjustments in my teaching load gave me the time to devote to this project. Counseling Department Chairperson J. Laurence Passmore, Division Director Leland Melvin, and the late dean of the School of Education, Richard L. Willey, were all involved in providing the necessary administrative support. The School of Education has employed as editors three women who have helped me make English out of my writing: Jane Angel, Linda Sanning, and Carole Gustafson. Doctoral fellows Cindy Williams, Steve Rumble, and Jim Mason did many of the boring but necessary bibliographic chores, while Lindy Hubert helped to find and then abstracted the licensing research studies. Departmental secretaries Rosie Coyle, Mary Alice Bemis, and Mary Lou Cooley somehow found time to transform my scribbling into readable print. The interlibrary loan staff at ISU's Cunningham Memorial Library, Carol Chapman, Mary Ann Phillips, and Karen Y. Stabler, was especially helpful, as was Marcella Guthrie at the circulation desk.

   Deb Oughton of the Illinois House Minority Leader's staff, Paul Pottinger, then director of the Center for the Study of the Professions, and Marvin J. Kolhoff of the General Electric Company helped me in getting started. The interest Norman Shealy and Dana Ullman took in my work was important to me. Laura Bakken's preparation of the final manuscript was quick and accurate. My daughter, Elizabeth Gross, helped with her clarification of procedural and substantive due process. Discussions with my wife, Julie McVay, were stimulating, supportive, and a reality check.

                                                                                                  S.J.G.

OF FOXES
AND HEN HOUSES

1

INTRODUCTION

AN OVERVIEW

Professional licensing as the solution to a problem has become worse than the problem it is said to address—the unwillingness and inability of the public to protect itself from harm and exploitation by incompetents and charlatans. The solution, proposed and essentially self-regulated by professionals themselves, has been to use the police power of the State to control the entry of persons to the ranks of those who serve the public. The resulting apparatus developed to maintain the enterprise not only has failed, it has failed at a heavy financial and social cost. At the same time, it serves to protect and enhance the income, security, status, and privilege of the self-appointed "protectors."

The consensus of research reviewed in this book is that licensing fails to assure its legitimate purpose of furthering competence and honesty in service. There is no convincing evidence from the research on occupational licensure of a tie between licensure and the quality of service (see chapter 8). Instead, the evidence, which is commonplace in the literatures of economics and sociology, indicates the purposes realized by such regulation have been to maintain and increase the incomes of those who are licensed and to provide them with career security (Benham, 1980). It does so by creating monopolies in particular services and by giving licensed professions the power of self-regulation. The result has been to validate occupations through legislation, to increase the cost of services by controlling the entry of practitioners, and to reinforce the public inclination to depend on experts by misleading them into believing they are being protected. The self-regulators have also been indifferent to the quacks and incompetents in their own ranks and have ignored legitimate demands for public accountability.

Liberman (1970), concerned about exploitation of the public, said that a significant number of professional practitioners are not deterred by "self-regulation," that the system of self-regulation is not conducive to such deterrence and that a "significant number" may be numerically or relatively small and yet be enough to call sharply into question the traditional means of controlling professional behavior . . . [so] some other form of control is necessary to protect the public and at the same time guard against an intellectual debasement of the place of the modern profession. [p. 282]

Mechanic (1976) referred to the problem as it applied to the medical profession, the occupation that has served as the model for other professions.

Unlike many other participants in complex organizations the physician has greater autonomy and a more profound mystique, and patients tend to be more dependent and trustful. Thus, it is especially important that mechanisms be developed that allow for recognition of existing conflicts and ways of adjudicating them so as to allow the work of the institution to go on while also protecting patients' rights. . . . [W]e have little evidence that self-policing is effective in dealing with such problems. [p. 55]

This issue arises at a time when health and helping professions are fighting with one another for the right to third-party payments and for a piece of a future national health insurance dollar. At the same time, the cost of services is escalating sharply, and the public is increasingly frustrated about the poor quality of health services. Greer et al. (1978) indicated that a widespread discontent existed.

Certainly there are many indications today that a large and influential body of notables and common citizens are disturbed by the imputed lack of accountability— read this irresponsibility—of the very public organs and publically certified professions which are supposed to care for their needs. . . . [There is] discontent with the terms of trade . . . [indicating] a strong belief among many that they are the victims of broken bargains—by doctors, hospitals, attorneys, and professors. [pp. 9-10]

The failure of professions to offer nondiscriminatory, innovative, low-cost, widely available, and competent professional service (Hogan, 1979a) and their profit from this failure while they are supposed to be protecting the public is an ethical question of the highest priority for modern professions. In short, we need to find ways to protect the public rather than professionals. The failure to address this question risks the credibility of professionals, the faith of the public, and the continued support of special privileges for professionals.

The search for an alternative to professional licensing begins with the understanding that licensing makes an important contribution to the above problems. Licensing supports the type of relationship between client and practitioner where the interests of the professional both oppose and gain dominance over those of the client. No matter how well intentioned many individual practitioners may be, despite their excellent training and continuing education and disregarding egalitarian sentiments and the personal characteristics essential to competence, it is the view here that the norms of professions, supported by the monopoly and autonomy generated by licensing, result in professionals' attitudes that too often lead to shoddy, impersonal, and dangerous service. Unfortunately, however, most people, including professionals, believe that professional licensing protects the public. Thus, they support the very apparatus that is the source of the exploitation and harm done by professionals to the public. Though the latent power in the client-professional relationship is with the client, professionals retain power by mystifying clients and withholding knowledge. Professionals will remain entrenched, unaware of their real impact, and resistant to change until such time as the public becomes properly suspicious of professionalism and calls into question the legitimacy of the licensing charter that supports professionals' special prerogatives. The best hope for change is to find ways to elicit the power of the public to protect itself. The alternatives proposed in this book introduce competition and accountability into the social structure of client-professional relationships. Here competition and accountability will be shown to create an increase in the actual protection of the public and a climate supportive of public self-protection.

PURPOSES OF CREDENTIALS: A POINT OF VIEW

A credential is a public testimony about an individual's qualifications—that the person is a good credit risk, that the person has a job, that the individual successfully completed a prescribed course of training, or that the person passed an examination of some sort. Credentials *inform* people who do not know the credentialed individual but who do know the public body that does the credentialing. Credentials are as old as organized social life. Seal rings, robes, and crowns served as insignia of authority in the past much as the cardinal's hat and the colonel's eagle does today. Our employment ID cards, drivers' licenses, credit cards, and club and association membership cards are our more prosaic modern-day equivalents.

These pieces of paper represent some of our many social roles, particularly those that would otherwise be too time consuming, too difficult, or too involving to explain. It is not possible, of course, to tell from credentials whether we would be a good friend or a good parent, but a credential will tell the librarian to whom a book should be charged. So credentials are matters of convenience. Their information saves time and energy. They are limited, however. They are not necessarily trusted. When I make a big purchase on my Master Charge or on my department store credit card, the sales clerk often calls to see if I really still have an account. Credentials sometimes say that people can do things they really cannot do. If the local business school sends over a typist and says the typist can type ninety words per minute, I expect that our personnel office will give the typist their own test.

If credentials only informed they would merely pose the problems of reliability and validity, but they pose more complex problems. A second purpose of credentialing inferred here is called *social control*. Certain kinds of information place people in social categories. Credentials sort people into valued and not-so-valued categories. Their membership in these categories may directly affect their opportunities and life choices. Credentials are used in this way to reduce the pool of employment applicants. An employer may require a high school diploma for a job that someone with sixth grade reading ability could do. The employer has less of a problem making a choice simply because there are fewer people to look at. It may upgrade the status of the job, and employers are more likely to think they get a more "classy" person, though "classy" does not necessarily relate to competence. In fact we know that the only thing school grades (thus school certificates) predict is subsequent school grades. School grades do not predict either competence or success in an occupation or profession. The result is that to-day the unemployment rate among young adults without a high school diploma is much greater than the rate among those with the diploma in spite of the fact that they often cannot be differentiated on the job. So credentials are serious business, involved, as they are, in both bread-and-butter and survival issues.

Another consequence of placing people into social categories is that they may be influenced to do particular, socially approved activities and not to do others. Let us return to the schooling example. Young people have been flooding our schools of business and engineering primarily because there has been a promise of jobs, security, and status. Many are enrolled in our universities, but they are uninterested in learning generally; uninterested even in the specific subjects of their study. They believe they are freely choosing to enroll in their particular courses of study, but they have been influenced to engage in an activity that is not intrinsically interesting to them. They believe, however, that they will get a job on the basis of having a college degree with a "good major"—a credential they (and most of the rest of us) are encouraged to think makes them somehow "better" than people who do not have that credential. The eventual impact of such thinking on their lives is to increase the likelihood of problems of motivation and adjustment on the job and in their social life with the attendant physiological and psychological symptoms of stress. Unfortunately, more of us face a choice between the stress that comes when you accept this credential mentality and the anxiety and uncertainty of not accepting it, of experiencing life on the margin of conventional society. On a broader front, our nation is deprived of the valuable human resources that would be available if our culture more actively encouraged young people to search and discover more freely.

Some of that control works specifically against the best interests of women. An example is the private secretary. Before the first world war private secretaries were mostly men and the men who held those jobs were often in training for an administrative position. This has not been the case for some time. Secretaries now are mostly women and they rarely gain administrative leadership appointments by being promoted from a secretary's rank. The job has not changed as much as its meaning as a social category has, to the detriment of life chances for many women.

Our credentials system also protects the people assigned to each social category. Recently a group of nurses were asked: "If you stripped away your distinctive caps, uniforms and badges, would your patients be able to distinguish your competence from that of other health service workers?" Naturally, they perceived this to be an anxiety-arousing question. The question exposed the core issue of personal competence, which our credentials mentality obfuscates. Consider the possibility of using other types of qualifications for school and occupational selection. Perhaps we would not get the jobs we hold now. Maybe we would be replaced by people who have some arbitrarily defined qualifications potentially unobtainable by us—younger people or people who are related to a politician or people who are native speakers of Spanish. This anxiety is the tip-off about the basic inequity of the system. If we have it working for us, we do not see this inequity. The people who have it working against them see it rather clearly. The type of academic training required to enter most occupations or the multiple-choice questions asked to examine "competence" make entry unobtainable for them, despite the irrelevance of such qualifications. This is how the system of credentialing is used as a social control device, keeping the "ins" in and the "outs" out. It is in this way the credentialing system, specifically the licensing of occupations, is at the crux of an inequitable occupational system.

TYPES OF REGULATION

There are various forms of occupational regulation and there are important distinctions among them. The focus here is on the type of regulation that employs the police power of the State. Activities such as malpractice suits by clients, credentialing of individuals by professional organizations, institutional accreditation, the Federal Trade Commission, and state and federal court decisions are all part of a general system of regulation. Through licensing, individuals are the direct beneficiaries of legislative actions. Licensing has been defined as

The granting by some competent authority of a right or permission to carry on a business or do an act which otherwise would be illegal. The essential elements of licensing involve the *stipulation of circumstances* under which permission to perform an otherwise prohibited activity may be granted—largely a legislative function; and the actual granting of the permission in specific cases—generally an administrative responsibility. [Council, 1952, p. 5]

The legislative authority for state governments to license has long been recognized. In a historic opinion, Justice Field, writing for the U.S. Supreme Court in 1889 in the case of a "physician" who did not have state approved credentials, held that:

It is undoubtedly the right of every citizen of the United States to follow any lawful calling, business or profession he may choose subject only to such restrictions as are imposed upon all persons of like age, sex and condition. . . . All may be pursued as sources of livelihood, some requiring years of study and great learning for their successful prosecution. . . . [T]he right to continue their prosecution is often of great value to the possessors, and cannot be arbitrarily taken from them. . . . But there is no arbitrary deprivation of such right where its exercise is not permitted because of a failure to comply with conditions imposed by the State for the protection of society. The power of the State to provide for the general welfare of its people authorizes it to prescribe all such regulations as in its judgment will secure or tend to secure them against the consequences of ignorance and incapacity as well as of deception and fraud. [*Dent* v. *State of West Virginia*, 1889, pp. 121-22]

In this opinion the court not only upheld the legitimacy of the use of police power to regulate occupations, it also confirmed that licensing validates an occupation as a property right and provided the rationale for licensing legislation. The courts have not interfered with this authority since that time unless a law has had no relationship to its legislative purpose or is arbitrary or capricious. They devote themselves instead to clarifying the boundaries between professions and reviewing the decisions of licensing agencies (Council, 1952).

Licensing is the generic term referring to all forms of state control over the right to perform specific activities. These means of control will be referred to here as *input regulation*, that is, the attempt to regulate by controlling who may carry on an activity rather than controlling the activity itself or assessing its consequences; in turn process and output regulation. There has been a good deal of confusion over teminology so three predominant forms of occupational licensing will be defined following Hogan's (1979a) usage as it seems to be more functional than others. He described three types of licensing: practice, title, and registration acts.

Practice Acts

Practice acts are the most restrictive and the most desired by professions. They have the following characteristics: (1) Authority is granted by a board or office of the State, a majority or entirety of whose members are usually representatives of the occupation it licenses. (2) Authority is granted solely to persons who have specifically defined qualifications (for example, age, residence, citizenship, character, approved educational program, and experience) and who can pass an entry examination that signifies the competence of the person to practice the occupation. (3) Only authorized persons are permitted to use particular occupational titles. Persons not so licensed are prevented from using such titles, thus restricting the use of titles or insignia. (4) They grant to authorized persons the authority to engage in defined tasks and prevent persons not so licensed from engaging in those tasks, thus mandating the boundaries of practice. By regulating the entry of persons into the practice of the tasks defined, the state creates a monopoly for the licensed occupation. By giving the occupation the power to regulate itself, the State permits the occupation's members to practice autonomously; in effect, the practitioners are their own judges of competent and ethical practice. Autonomy, however, is not characteristic of all occupations licensed by a practice act. Those in some occupations (for example, nursing, physician's assistant) are required to be subordinate to practitioners of other occupations in actual practice as well as subordinate to the dominant occupation on state licensing boards. Others (for example, school teachers) practice in institutional settings and are subject to administrators' decisions about their activities.

Some professions such as medicine have rather wide scopes of practice. This poses a problem for other health professions. Without their own licensure act or a specific exemption in the medical practice act, other health professionals would be prohibited from practice. Christoffel (1982) also pointed out that licensed practitioners are permitted by many state laws "to delegate some functions and duties, provided they are carried out under the control and supervision of the delegator" (p. 82). Technological change frequently is ahead of what these acts permit, making for problems as well as social arrangements that ignore the restrictive provisions of the law.

It is the practice act that is considered to be the pinnacle for the professions. The legal grant of power that makes the unauthorized practice a criminal matter not only dubs the occupation with a legitimizing grace, it gives the occupation control over who does the work of the occupation, how it is done, what is done, and, in effect, to whom it is done. It is this type of licensing that most abuses the public trust, for which we find little justification and that is the subject for our concern in this book. Some writers (Friedman, 1962, among others) have used the term *licensing* or *compulsory licensing* to refer to practice acts. Since so many persons also use licensing to describe all state-sponsored occupational regulation, its use will be restricted here to this latter generic sense.

Title Acts

Title acts are often referred to as certification or as voluntary or partial licensing. They grant authority to use an occupational title to persons who meet particular qualifications as determined by the occupation's self-regulated board. Because title acts do not restrict the authority to engage in particular tasks, they permit competition. They are often described as voluntary or permissive because they do not forbid the practice of an occupation by nonlicensed persons (for example, accountants). Instead, they restrict the use of a particular occupational title (for example, certified public accountant) prohibit the use of designating insignia by nonmembers of the resricted occupation (for example, CPA). Title acts are similar to practice acts in that a self-regulating board determines which qualifications are suitable and an entry examination is used to establish presumed competency. The practitioner's monopoly is reduced by the fact that non-licensed practitioners are permitted to consult with the public.

Registration Acts

Registration acts are the least restrictive form of state-controlled occupational regulation. Registration is usually a listing of persons who perform certain tasks and may be mandatory or voluntary. They ordinarily do not require any prior showing of qualifications and ordinarily do not impose an entry test of competence. They grant authority to engage in particular tasks only. Practitioners on a registry may have their permit to practice revoked or suspended if they violate stipulated practice standards. The state agency administering the law is usually not linked to the occupational group it regulates. Since there are no special entry restrictions, competition is maximized. The absence of self-regulating boards avoids state support for occupational autonomy.

Some Other Forms of Regulation

With Hogan (1979a) and Roemer (1974), the term *certification* will be used to refer to the credentialing of competency by private associations. The American Dietetic Association certifies dietitians when they award them the R.D. The specialty boards of the AMA certify physicians specializing in radiology, internal medicine, and so on. Government is not involved in the direct act of credentialing, though it may require the use of a certified person (for example, registered dietitians in nursing homes) in the absence of licensing arrangements for the occupation.

Accreditation ordinarily refers to the activities of both public and private agencies and associations, which determine whether a training or educational program meets predetermined standards. Accreditation may also be stipulated in state-controlled occupational regulation and legislation authorizing public services. Regional accrediting associations, though privately sponsored and cooperatively funded by member institutions, accredit secondary schools and higher education institutional programs generally. Professional associations may accredit specific educational programs in their field. A strong component of accreditation is the concept of periodic reassessment of programs which may occur on five- or ten-year cycles, for example. It is a program, not a person, that is being accredited. This is important because individual credentialing often requires accreditation of the training program preparing the person. Also, individuals may use the fact that this training was accredited as an informal credential as our doctors and lawyers do when they hang their diplomas from their accredited institutions on their waiting room walls.

Institutional licensure refers to the extension of facility licensure (for example, hospitals) to include personnel. The employing institution is responsible for the development of procedures pertinent to job definition, review of job classification, and training and supervision requirements (Roemer, 1974). It may be done by a state, county, municipality, or the federal government. This was recommended as a way out of the dilemma caused by the restrictive legal definitions of individual licensure, which prevents personnel from performing tasks identified as belonging to another occupation. If a nurse prescribed medication for a patient, to use an obvious example, the nurse would be stepping out of the prescribed role of a nurse under individual licensure and would be potentially liable for criminal action as well as a malpractice suit. But in a licensed institution, a nurse could have a job description that would permit prescribing medication. The interest in this alternative has receded because the professions involved are politically powerful enough to block an alternative that circumvented individual licensure.

Still other forms of credentialing find their way into discussions of regulation, particularly when attention turns to agencies or training institutions rather than to individuals. *Approval* occurs when an agency is reviewed generally on the basis of past performance and specific criteria and may thus be identified as rendering a service worthy of some notice. A *charter* establishes an institution's corporate identity under the laws of the state permitting the institution to award degrees or offer a service, for profit or not for profit. *Recognition* is another review process that is service specific. An agency may have a function assessed that is related to but not basic to its primary purpose. It seeks recognition with the intent of identifying this function to the public as being carried out with integrity. (The Study, 1979).

GAINING THE LEGISLATION

It is easy to see why the area of occupational licensing has become a tangle of regulations, jurisdictions, and agencies and an arena of conflict between public and private interests by examining the process by which such legislation wins passage. It is important to note in passing that these struggles should not be viewed in isolation. They are the surface manifestation of a variety of political and social forces striving for dominance. This will be discussed in some detail in chapters 3, 4, and 5.

Friedman (1962) described the overall process of gaining licensing legislation as the interaction between concentrated vested interests on the one hand and an amorphous, dispersed public interest on the other.

People in the same trade, like barbers or physicians, all have an intense interest in the specific problems of this trade and are willing to devote considerable energy to doing something about them. On the other hand, those of us who use barbers at all, get barbered infrequently and spend only a minor fraction of our income in barber shops. Our interest is casual. Hardly any of us are willing to devote much time going to the legislature in order to testify against the inequity of restricting the practice of barbering. [p. 143].

The process of gaining licensing legislation usually begins with an occupational group, professional society, trade association, or labor union interested in the legislation. Few licensing laws have departed from this scenario. The group to be regulated becomes the driving force for licensing, hoping to achieve goals through licensing that they have been unable to attain on their own. The group will then draft a proposed statute that defines the occupation and activities, sets up a board to govern the occupation, authorizes the board to conduct examinations, provides for an administrative apparatus and a fee structure, and defines penalties for violation of the act. National professional associations have drawn up model acts which they then send to their state associations for implementation. Ordinarily, these groups will begin with mild regulations so as not to arouse opposition while laying their claim to an area of practice or service. It has been the history of these arrangements for them to increase in their restrictiveness with the passage of time.

The next step is to find a sponsor—a member of the legislature disposed in favor of the bill, willing to campaign for it, and who has sufficient finesse and respect in the legislature to enable the legislator to win the behind-the-scenes committee fights that torpedo most bills entered onto legislature dockets. The occupational group then puts its resources into support for the bill; letter-writing campaigns, testifying before legislative committees, and "buttonholing" individual legislators. Ordinarily, the "protection of the public" argument will be used with some emphasis on the potential "danger" of the activity in the hands of the uninformed and unscrupulous. Usually, the bill follows a torturous journey toward a legislative decision attempting to avoid being ignored by the legislators on one hand and to avoid too much publicity on the other hand. Too much publicity might incite a challenge from those who potentially would be harmed by the legislation: prospective entrants, consumer groups, labor organizations, or employers. As Haberfield et al. (1978) indicate, they are usually successful.

Unfortunately, little aid is offered the legislature to insure that it hears all sides of the issue before making [the] decision. . . . Ideally, the airing of conflicting views through lobbyists and counter-lobbyists can indicate the possible strengths, weaknesses and long-term effects of a measure. However, in the case of a licensing bill there will be relatively few voices of dissent heard. [p. A-18]

After the law has been passed there is little likelihood, as has been indicated previously, that the courts would interfere with this use of police powers. Though states have been cautioned by the courts not to use police powers as a pretext to interfere with private business or occupation, the courts have been reluctant to get involved if there is any rational connection at all between the law and the public interest objectives. In fact, Payne's (1977) search of the legal literature unearthed only two instances when the U.S. Supreme Court invalidated state statutes as improper.

THE DILEMMA OF REGULATION

It helps when considering the problem of regulation to decide from what perspective it is viewed. Abraham Lincoln described one such situation. "The shepherd drives the wolf from the sheep's throat, for which the sheep thanks the shepherd as his liberator, while the wolf denounces him for the same act as the destroyer of liberty" (Peter, 1977, p. 208). The essential dilemma of regulation can be understood by considering that the shepherd also keeps the sheep in bondage, exploits the sheep for its wool, and eventually kills it for the same purpose the wolf intended—for its meat. Dilemmas are situations in which difficulties are present no matter what is done. Milgrom (1978), writing about the regulation of dentists, made a statement that might be applied to most professionals. "There are serious problems in asking dentists to regulate themselves, and even worse problems in not asking them to do so" (p. 115). Others might put it in the reverse way, arguing that the more serious problems occur when professionals are asked to regulate themselves. Either way, regulation appears to have two basic characteristics. First, it assumes vulnerability and helplessness on the part of the public. Second, it poses the problem: "Who guards the guardian?"

Vulnerability

The vulnerability of the consumer is assumed in economic theory. The protection offered to buyers and sellers in a competitive situation, through the existence of alternatives, functions only in general and in the long run. In the short run, "the existence of alternatives does not prevent acts such as violence, fraud, misrepresentation, breach of contract, intentionally malevolent action or appropriations of trademarks" (Barron, 1966, p. 641). The existence of alternatives may offer some protection to buyers who go from seller to seller prior to buying, and buyers who will be wiser the *next* time, once burned by a seller. But there are situations according to Barron that cannot be rectified or for which compensation cannot be found.

One does not rectify death from the consumption of adulterated foods or the performance of an operation with a contaminated scalpel; nor is blindness from drinking methyl alcohol sold as grain alcohol easily corrected. . . . [G]eneral laws governing such areas as sanitation, purity of foods, and industrial safety are not sufficient to protect ignorant buyers. [p. 642]

The economic rationale for licensing individuals then is "to insure that buyers can make choices among sellers who meet some minimum standard of competence—the 'no second choice' argument" (Barron, 1966, p. 643). Blair and Kaserman (1980) distinguish three types of characteristics for commodities. *Search* characteristics can be ascertained prior to purchase. *Experience* characteristics can be determined with use. *Credence* characteristics cannot be evaluated even with normal use. "Services rendered by professionals are strongly marked by credence characteristics. . . . The potential for undetected quality reductions stems from asymmetric information sets. The seller knows, the buyer does not" (p. 186).

The assumption that the consumer is vulnerable and helpless, though a constant factor in economic theory, is questioned here, as is its corollary that the responsibility for consumer protection belongs to society as a whole. The very perception of the problem of vulnerability may be a function of viewing it from the standpoint of the professional. If instead, for example, theorists assumed that consumers have a special awareness of their own needs and a general interest in maximizing them, ways may be considered to enhance the operation of these factors in economic transactions. Reversing informational imbalances is one tactic characteristic of the self-help and self-care movements. This perspective is the basis for the quest for alternatives to licensing discussed in chapter 9.

Who Guards the Guardian?

The fox guarding the hen house poses a conflict of interest that is especially difficult because professionals have both special competence and their own interests. Krause (1977) pointed to the danger of co-optation when there is a dependence on expertise.

If a process is highly technical, and yet of basic importance to a society, then experts must be enlisted to supervise and guard the process in the interests of the public. But they must guard their fellow experts (perhaps personally known to them) and often these are members of exactly the same profession. The public does not have the option of ignoring its need for expert consultation, nor can it ignore the possibility that experts in the regulatory role might work in the interests of the regulated rather than in the general interest. [p. 275]

Whether and how any society can find ways to involve professionals and restrain their inclinations to act in their own self-interest will be an underlying theme throughout this book.

Several means have been devised to control the inclination of professionals to act in their own self-interest but these pose additional problems. Applying the rational methods of bureaucracy has the intention of reducing subjectivity and inefficiency, both expressions of self-interest. Mechanic (1979), however, pointed out that regulations may be subverted through an overemphasis on rationality.

Most rules are easily subverted in practice; when regulations are imposed, efforts are often devoted to meeting their bureaucratic requirements without major impact on behavior. . . . [I]n considering imposing possible controls on the service sector, it is necessary to weigh the magnitude of the problems and the likely gains achieved through regulation against the costs of imposing further bureaucratic rules. [p. 105]

Consequently, effective regulation must find a middle ground between need and the possibility of gain.

A related question has to do with the scope of regulation. What should be covered and what should be left alone for the operation of natural social processes? Regulations can be too inclusive or too restrictive. Unrealistically broad or too restrictive a regulation may have the effect of driving people to use illegal services, to perform the services themselves, or to do without the services altogether. This occurs because restrictive regulation tends to reduce the amount of services available and drive up the price of what is left.

Regulations may also be too complex. Krause (1977) pointed to the health field where there are

many different protoregulatory agencies . . . each of which has a "piece of the action": e.g., licensing boards judge fitness to practice; hospital accreditation and licensing agencies approve health settings; and state insurance commissions, rate-setting commissioners, or the federal government approve insurance rates for third-party payers. . . . [T]hough there is one field (health care) there are many regulatory agencies, usually not working together, and sometimes even working at cross purposes. [p. 277]

It is no wonder that the purposes of regulations may become lost in a maze and that issues of efficiency, fairness, consumer protection, and accountability are not raised. Nonetheless, the problems and dilemmas of regulation have appeared important for many to solve since the alternatives of state ownership on the one hand or deregulation on the other have been perceived as far worse. This book reports on the various attempts to find that middle ground.

2

WHY REGULATE?

Licensing is a means of regulating occupations under the police powers of the State. The question "Why regulate?" is answered by a discussion of the purposes of licensing. Then the case against licensing is detailed following a statement of the six major arguments against it.

THE PURPOSES OF LICENSING

Licensing is justified as having either a public welfare or a professional welfare purpose. We shall begin with the public welfare rationale as this is the one usually heard when occupations argue the merits of their cases before state legislatures.

Public Welfare Purposes

The much discussed purpose of licensing is to protect the public from harm and fraud at the hands of incompetent and unethical practitioners. Since licensing is enacted under the police powers of the State, public welfare is the primary justification offered for measures that ensure competency and honesty in services offered to the public. The argument is that without some type of regulation the citizenry would suffer irreparable physical harm, emotional injury, or financial loss at the hands of practitioners whose lack of skill, knowledge, or ethics makes them unable or unwilling to foresee or forestall the commission of hurt to those they are supposed to serve. By establishing and maintaining quality standards for practitioners through selection, examination, and disciplining of licensees, licensing agencies prevent the unscrupulous and the unqualified from practice and provide a means by which aggrieved members of the public may gain redress for received hurt.

Lieberman (1970) detailed the kinds of activity that have been used to justify licensing.

(1) [A]ctivity which if negligently performed may lead to death or serious bodily injury; (2) activity which may result in deprivation of legal rights; (3) activity resulting in defective craftsmanship of an objective nature (e.g., watchmaking); (4) activity resulting in defective craftsmanship of a subjective nature (e.g., photography); (5) activity by those who receive money in advance or those who do not have a fixed place of business; and (6) activity involving a fiduciary trust the breach of which can lead to serious psychological or economic injury [p. 246]

The reasons why licensing is believed to be necessary have to do with human nature and the conditions of modern society. Three reasons have been mentioned as necessitating some form of regulation of service givers. These include the "lack of information," "third party," and "society knows best" rationales.

First, the poor ability of consumers to distinguish the competent from the incompetent practitioner and the honorable from the unethical practitioner raises the vulnerability question. Can the public be protected from its own ignorance and credulity? The information needed by consumers is often difficult, costly, and time-consuming to obtain and when available often requires sophistication to interpret correctly. The intense specialization in all professional fields has made the information all the more esoteric. Mechanic (1979) has said "Professional-client relationships, particularly in medical care, are characterized by great inequality in knowledge" (p. 42). The consumer also has great difficulty in comparing professional services prior to consuming them (Payne, 1977). In an anonymous urban society, information about a professional's reputation is not passed from neighbor to friend to relative as it might be in a more closely knit society.

A corollary economic justification for regulation is related to the cost of information about practitioners' competency. According to Leffler (1978),

costly information will also tend to directly shift the equilibrium distribution of quality supplied towards lower quality as information costs rise. This results from a lower demand for high quality practitioners due to the difficulty of locating and evaluating high quality suppliers. [p. 173]

Regulating these market forces via licensing is justified especially if other jurisdictions impose regulations. A "bad money" theory is promulgated whereby, like unstable currency, lower quality practitioners are driven from more strictly regulated jurisdictions and professions to less strictly regulated jurisdictions and professions (Swain, 1975; Tochen, 1978).

The mystification created by an authoritative voice amongst ignorance permits placebo or "hocus pocus" effects (Leffler, 1978). These effects are enhanced, though, by the patient's exceedingly high expectations for the practitioner. This results in people believing they are being treated competently and honestly when they may not be. Ignorance may also result in disdain for authority, producing the opposite effect whereby people believe they are being treated incompetently and fraudulently when in fact they are not. Etither way, "hocus pocus" distorts the judgments of some consumers. Leffler reported that surveys of physicians show that more than 35 percent of money paid for physicians' services were for placebo ministrations.

Judgments may be distorted anyway because consumers are usually in some sort of crisis when they consult a professional. This causes them to be especially vulnerable to the expert they hope might rescue them from the crisis. They are vulnerable to both those who would and those who would not take advantage of their confusion or naivete. Mechanic (1979) has said, "In periods of high stress in which decisions must be made quickly, persons often reveal a pattern of hyper vigilance that is associated with cognitive constriction, perseveration, and disrupted thought processes and that interferes significantly with rational choice" (p. 42). The net result of these factors is to raise serious questions about whether consumers can be competent to act in their own best interests when judging the skill, knowledge, or ethical standards of a professional service giver. Mechanic indicated that patients tended to make judgments on factors that are not particularly good predictors of the physician's knowledge or diagnostic skills: "whether the physician communicates a personal interest in the patient, whether he listens carefully, whether he shows a sympathetic concern and provides feedback, and whether he appears to know what he is doing" (p. 43). It is interesting to note that these are factors that are associated with improvements in health of patients.

A second reason given for regulating service givers is the so-called third-party or epidemic effect. The argument is, given the consumers' poor ability to judge quality, they may make a poor judgment about a service, which produces harmful effects not just for themselves but also for others. The example often cited is of the consumer who chooses a "lower quality" health service practitioner who is unable to distinguish a functional from an organic malady or one organic malady from another. Such a practitioner may not diagnose and treat a communicable disease, thus permitting it to be spread to others, innocent and uninvolved in this transaction. In another field entirely, the editor of *The Journal of Accountancy* argues similarly for the regulation of auditors (who sign the financial statements which purport to represent accurately the monetary state of a company) since "third parties who rely on financial statements do not usually have an opportunity to exercise judgment in the selection of the auditor and may be seriously hurt if the statements are misleading" (Legislation, 1960, p. 28).

Martin (1980) pointed out that this effect, called an "externality" by economists, might also emerge from the sale of low quality (read that unlicensed) services offered by plumbers, electricians, or barbers. This third-party effect is thus a natural consequence of the consumer's difficulty in making an appropriate individual judgment of quality.

A third reason for regulating service givers, the "society knows best" theory, also discounts the ability of individual consumers to know what is best for themselves. This argument contends that even in the unlikely event that people have perfect knowledge of past, present, and future, they still would not be the best judges of what is in their own welfare; society knows better. This view relies heavily on the growth of scientific knowledge and the thesis that individuals are overly optimistic in evaluating the expected results of their actions (Moore, 1961). Leffler (1978) describes the assumption here that "individuals underestimate the risks from consuming low quality services, but the same individuals correctly anticipate the expected results for the rest of society" (p. 175). This is similar to the often reported disparity between the judgments individuals make about the poor quality of America's health services and the satisfaction the same individuals report about the quality of service they receive from their own personal physician.

In evaluating these reasons for licensing, Moore (1961) pointed out that licensing of occupations is more likely: (1) the greater the variety in the quality of service furnished by practitioners; (2) the greater the possibility of harm accruing from poor service; (3) the greater the skill needed to evaluate the furnished service; and (4) the less exposure the consumer has to the practitioner. Concern for the improvement of consumer choice, according to both Moore (1961) and Leffler (1978), argues in favor of title acts and registration under a "lack of information" rationale and in favor of practice acts under the "third party" and "society knows best" rationales. Practice acts give no more information to the consumer than title acts and are no more effective against fraud than registration acts, according to Moore (1961). Title and registration acts do preserve freedom of choice for the consumer. The existence of low-quality and potentially harmful service, however, poses the possibility that social costs are greater than private costs in some instances (that is, that others besides the service buyer are harmed by the buyer's purchase decision). Practice acts that control who may offer service are justified by this rationale. Moore (1961) believed that "only in the case of a few occupations—such as physicians, veterinarians, and pharmacists—is it possible to argue that social costs are greater than private costs" (p. 110). He cautioned, however, that when less well-trained persons were prevented from practicing, the average price of service increased, raising the possibility that some persons will decide to forego purchasing the service. To justify practice acts, he indicated, it is necessary "to argue as well that the harm done through purchasing from 'incompetent' practitioners is greater than the possible harm alone through not purchasing the service at all" (p. 110).

Professional Welfare

The imposition of control over occupations through licensing has for the most part not been thrust upon unwilling occupations but rather has been

eagerly sought by them. Gellhorn (1960) identified the following occupations on which licensing had been imposed to halt demonstrated abuses.
They include: saloon keeper, ship's officer, prize fighter, securities dealer,
private detective, and longshoreman. White (1979b) discussed the imposition of licensing on X-ray technicians and clinical laboratory personnel,
these efforts being led by bureaucrats with little observable public clamor.
Otherwise, members of occupations themselves have pursued their own
licensing. Two traditional reasons appear to explain this circumstance.
First, the creation of a competitive advantage through a state-ordained
monopoly of a particular service (via a practice act) leads to a heightened
income and job security for those meeting the special qualifications. Second,
licensing has become one of the characteristics attributed to a profession
(Goode, 1960). Consequently, occupations in pursuit of dignity and prestige
have sought licensing to enhance their public images. Witness the statement
made at a public hearing before the California Senate Committee on Business
and Professions in 1967 in behalf of social work: "Social work has certain
. . . reasons for needing regulation. These are: to establish a true and dignified public image of social work and to increase public confidence and understanding of social work" (Haberfield et al., 1978, p. A-12).

That licensing accomplishes these goals for occupations is attested to by the
widespread emulation of licensed professionals. The pressure from nonprofessional occupations to become professional has been particularly evident
recently as a result of specialization in health occupations, as we shall see in
chapter 3. Gerstl and Jacobs (1976) observed that the mystique of the
professional was considered socially useful for so many purposes that there
has been no consideration that it could be a liability. Haberfield et al. (1978)
reported the statement made by a representative of the California State
Department of Mental Hygiene before the California Senate Interim
Committee on Licensing Business and Professions in 1955. When asked about
the department's attitude toward the proposed licensing of psychiatric
technicians, the representative replied, "recognition should be given to this
vast field of operators so that they might be duly licensed *so that their
profession might be recognized and receive the dignity to which it is entitled"*
(p. A-12).

The same committee heard an attorney for the California Medical
Association justify licensing for the purposes of career security: "It seems to
me in the professions where many years of education and experience is [sic]
demanded before one may freely practice, that *the group is justly entitled to
governmental protection against encroachment by the untrained and
unskilled"* (p. A-11).

Dual Effects?

A third reason why professionals have pursued their own licensing has
emerged in the last decade. Actually, it is a combination of the first two

reasons. In chapter 3 we detail the war among the helping professions to monopolize for some, or to protect for others, the right to offer psychotherapy to the public and for occupations to gain status as reputable care givers (for example, counselors). Confusion abounds as the public hears concern about its welfare, but the consequences of licensing appear to benefit practitioners. The public hears about "diploma mill degrees," "sexual abuse by unlicensable therapists," and "psychotic episodes precipitated by incompetent diagnosis and treatment." Experts announce that only they—those with the highest academic qualifications, intensive long-term training, and who respect an ethical code—should be allowed to offer psychotherapy to the public. Tennov (1975) believed that these scare tactics gave a false picture

of a field in which nobody really knows much about what goes on, or what training is appropriate, or how to distinguish a good therapist from a poor one. . . . The issue is limiting the right to practice to those who have undergone extensive training when the relevance of that training to effectiveness is dubious, when there is a greater demand for services than can be met by those who would meet licensing requirements, and when experts have recommended the adoption of techniques pioneered by non-professionals. [pp. 140-41]

The legitimate purposes of licensing are compelling. People indeed have difficulty in protecting themselves. Yet a system that appears to operate to benefit those who serve the public raises questions about whether it can accomplish what its proponents say it can, and if it cannot, about what kind of system, if any, could do so. It may also be asked whether licensed professionals are a national resource that needs to be protected. Finally, is there justification for using the constitutionally guaranteed police powers of the State in this realm of our social and economic life? In this regard, Whitesel (1977) offered the "dual effects" theory whereby regulation at best may be understood to protect both the public and those in an occupation. In this case, with the balance of freedom of choice and the public good, legislators are left with estimating the degree to which one can or should overbalance the other.

THE CASE AGAINST LICENSING

The arguments against licensing were identified in the now classic *Occupational Licensing Regulation in the States* (Council, 1952). These are quoted below to introduce the six basic arguments, followed by a general explication of each argument with supporting data included wherever appropriate.

It is important to note that these social costs or adverse effects on the public welfare are considered "worth it" in some quarters because of the belief that licensing is essential to the public interest. These inevitable consequences of regulation, therefore, are considered by some to be unfortunate but necessary. Ultimately, the public decides at what degree of social cost licensing is no longer "worth it."

Artificial Scarcity

First, licensing agencies may limit the number of entrants to any occupation by establishing unduly restrictive experience and educational requirements. This tends to create an artificial scarcity of trained men. [Council, 1952, p. 3]

The examples of entry restraints often cited refer to physicians. Makofsky (1977) charged that a politically and economically powerful medical profession had been able to restrict the number of physicians available for primary practice to less than half the number needed for adequate treatment. Krause (1977) reported in the same vein that the number of medical school graduates was held constant from the 1930s to the 1960s despite rapid population growth. Carlson (1970) reported a steady per capita decline in physicians. Current licensure laws (Alford, 1975; Freidson, 1970) permit physicians an extensive monopoly and autonomy which, in turn, are the sources of their power over medical school enrollments. Professional control over licensing boards permits the manipulation of the examination pass rate. There is a good deal of evidence (discussed in the next section) that the consequence of this manipulation is to reduce competition and to increase income. Hogan (1979a) reported that "pass rates on licensing examinations in many occupations vary inversely with the level of unemployment (p. 267). The use of citizenship, prior local residency, lack of a criminal record, and the vague "good moral character" have questionable value in protecting the public but do reduce competition.

The most obvious effects may be seen in the shortages of medical personnel in rural areas and among the urban poor (Hogan, 1979a). Freidson (1970) integrated the themes of shortage, undue restriction on entry, and control when he charged that organized medicine

asserts its control over the performance of medical work at the same time its practitioners are too few to perform the work. It refuses to allow members of other occupations to perform such work except in a position of subordination from which they can gain little satisfaction. It insists on its jurisdiction over everything related to that vague word "health," including that vast, undifferentiated problem called "mental illness" for which neither medicine nor any other discipline has demonstrated any consistently effective therapeutic solution. [p. 235]

Carlson (1970) indicated that shortages

are exacerbated by licensure laws. To be employed in the health field, personnel must fit into licensure categories which vary from state to state but are uniformly restrictive in their application. Legal boundaries around manpower categories have led ineluctably to suboptimal utilization by precluding the matching of skills with the tasks to be performed. Entry barriers created by such laws restrict the supply of new manpower in the health field. State to state variations in licensure laws restrain interstate mobility, which possibly would alleviate the shortages caused by maldistribution. [p. 856]

Roemer's (1973) study of health personnel regulation in seven countries suggested that "legal definitions of scope of practice, by circumscribing the functions that may be performed, may restrict productivity of personnel, which could be expanded safely" (p. 234). By defining professional practice, licensing makes illegal (in some cases) and subject to malpractice action (in others) the delegation of identified functions from physicians to paramedical personnel. This locks physicians into performing tasks that they may be less capable of handling than are their assistants. With rapid technological change, physicians may be "supervising" personnel who know far more about their tasks than do the physicians.

By far the most insidious effect of licensing emanates from the fact that "current licensure laws in the health field virtually define the physicians as the consumer's only legitimate, primary contact with the health care system" (Alford, 1975, p. 196). Given the undersupply and maldistribution of physicians and the restrictions on who may be consulted, many consumers are not free to choose their health care providers. The relationship with consumers tends to take on much more of a "take-it-or-leave-it" character than would be true were there more choices open to consumers. The physician is less willing to invest the time and energy in negotiating the terms of the relationship and to attend to consumer preferences and demands to educate patients and is more likely to "dump" especially demanding patients (Freidson, 1970).

The effects of unduly restrictive licensing requirements can be generalized for other licensed occupations to the extent that they exert a similar degree of control over professional entry procedures. Though few professions have the degree of control maintained by the medical profession, the example of the medical profession is not irrelevant as it is the model of professionalization generally aspired to by other professions. In other words, the future of continued professionalization is evident now through an examination of its operation in medicine. Collins (1979) concluded that

the model of professional organizations has been widely emulated outside of the traditional professional occupations. . . . [T]he elaboration of educational credentials, licensing procedures, and other formally monopolistic structures is found not only among dentists, librarians, and teachers, but also spreads to accountants, medical technicians, morticians, social workers, and business administrators, and into the traditional skilled crafts of the construction and household repairs occupations. [p. 178]

Monopoly

Second, by creating monopoly conditions through erection of barriers to admission and through non-competitive standards of practice, they may raise prices and restrain competition to a degree detrimental to the people as a whole. [Council, 1952, pp. 3-4]

There is a considerable amount of evidence that the immediate consequences of monopolistic entry restrictions and intraprofessional restraints on competition are to raise prices, thus raising the income of practitioners and providing them with job insurance. Economists have long been interested in the effect that entry restrictions have on prices and income. The theory used is that licensing by restricting entry decreases supply. Assuming that demand remains the same, prices to the consumer and income to the practitioner are increased as the result of competition for the reduced supply. In addition, the costs of obtaining the license are passed on to the consumer. This research has special meaning today because of the centrality of the cost of services in skyrocketing health care costs. The price of services also has an effect on availability, pricing some consumers out of the market. In this way there is an implied relationship between higher costs and lowered quality.

Pfeffer (1974) reviewed the research and concluded "Occupational licensing operates to restrict entry and enhance occupational incomes" (p. 104). He reported relationships (a) between the enactment of licensing laws and the decline in the numbers of training institutions and trainees, (b) between the control of competitive behavior among professionals and an oversupply of professionals (to maintain the illusion of professional dominance), and (c) between the restrictiveness of a profession and its independence from local economic conditions. Moore (1961) found that restrictions on entry benefit the practitioners in the field at the time the restrictions are imposed. He reported the imposition of citizenship requirements for regulated occupations in Illinois in 1939, for example, at the time when there was a large influx of trained practitioners from Europe.

Payne (1977) reported on a study which found that "approximately one-half of the considerable income difference between licensed professionals and unlicensed nonprofessionals was the result of the greater difficulty of attaining entry (imposed by licensure requirements) into those professions" (p. III-5). Higher prices are the result of the limitations on the supply of qualified practitioners as well as the costs of obtaining the licensed credential which are passed on to the consumer (Tochen, 1978).

Haberfield, et al. (1978) detailed these immediate effects:

(1) reduced occupational opportunity and buying power for individuals; (2) increased unemployment among the population at large and among certain minority or disadvantaged groups in particular; (3) higher consumer prices in an artificially

constructed market place; [and] (4) a decreased range of consumer choice among goods and services. [p. A-24]

The particular means of controlling entry is the manipulation of the examination pass rate. Cohen and Mike (1974) and Krause (1977) report the practice of permitting foreign physicians to practice in chronic-disease and mental hospitals—either ignoring citizenship requirements or lowering examination passing level for those who would work in less desirable settings or in geographical areas of high need. Holen (1965) used census data for physicians, lawyers, and dentists and found that states which had high failure rates were associated with high practitioner average incomes. Benham, Maurizi and Reder (1968) found a positive relationship between failure rates and income for dentists but not for physicians. Maurizi's study (1974) hypothesized a relationship between an increasing number of new applicants per licensed practitioner and a higher failure rate for new applicants. Reviewing data collected by the Council of State Governments on 18 occupations for the years 1940 and 1950 he found that a 10 percent increase in the number of new applicants per licensed practitioner generated "a decrease in pass rate varying from 1 percent to 10 percent depending on the occupation" (p. 412). He also found that a "10 percent increase in average practitioner incomes produces up to a 10 percent decrease in the pass rate" (p. 412). He concluded, "the power of licensing boards is often used to prolong the period of higher incomes resulting from increases in excess demand for the services of the occupation in question and that the instrument then used to accomplish this purpose is alteration of the pass rate on the licensure examination" (p. 412). Pfeffer (1974) also used Council of State Government data to compute correlations "between occupational income and the proportion passing the examinations or obtaining licenses, controlling for state median income" (p. 108). He found significant negative relationships (high income and low pass rate) for accountants ($-.317$, $p<.10$), attorneys ($-.616$, $p<.05$), and dentists ($-.588$, $p<.005$). Correlations for pharmacists, barbers, and real estate agents were not significant. Carroll and Gaston (1979a), using data from the National Association of Real Estate License Law Officials and the census, found a significant negative association ($p<.01$) between real estate brokers' pass rate and their median earnings. Pass rate investigation, they concluded, revealed the income enhancement role of licensing clearly at work.

Carroll and Gaston (1979b), following a procedure initiated by Maurizi (1974) on data for 1940 and 1950, used 1974 data to compare examination pass rates according to the number of licensed practitioners in a state. They found significant negative relationships for accountants ($p<.01$), architects ($p<.05$), barbers ($p<.05$), practical nurses ($p<.01$), registered nurses ($p<.05$), pharmacists ($p<.01$), physicians ($p<.01$), and plumbers ($p<.05$). Occupations where a significant relationship was not found included attorneys, podiatrists, chiropractors, cosmotologists, dental hygienists, dentists, embalmers, funeral directors, optometrists, osteopaths, physical therapists, psychologists, real estate agents, sanitarians, tree experts and veterinarians. They concluded that the tendency to use examination pass rates to respond to excess demand was more pronounced than in 1940 and 1950.

Benham and Benham (1975) studied the relationship between professional control of an eye care occupation and the price of eyeglasses. Comparing the prices between restrictive and nonrestrictive states they found prices to be from 25 percent to 40 percent higher where there was greater professional control. Sheppard (1978) studied twelve common dental services comparing the price in states which permit reciprocity (low restriction) to states which do not permit reciprocity (high restriction). He found that for eleven of these services fees were significantly higher (p < .05) in states which did not permit reciprocity. Three services (periodic oral exams, dental prophylaxis and tooth removals) which accounted for more than one-half of all services performed by U.S. dentists were 8.5 to 17.9 percent more expensive in states not permitting reciprocity. Fees were also substantially greater in such states for more complicated root canal (9.8 percent), gold inlay (7.9 percent), gold crown (6.2 percent), and dental bridge procedures (7.7 percent). The only service where prices were comparable (denture repair) accounted only for one-half of one percent of all dental visits. Begun (1980) found "legislated professionalism," which included four restrictive variables, was positively associated with higher prices for optometric examinations. Three of the variables (required continuing education, prohibition of optician price advertising and restricted mercantile location) were related to higher prices while prohibition of optometrist price advertising was not.

The research on the economic costs of licensing makes the point clearly that although licensing is not always associated with higher incomes, where it is associated with a barrier to competition (restrictions on reciprocity, fee schedules and examination pass rates) it tends to increase the incomes of practitioners. The relationship between licensing and the price of services appears even firmer.

Though there is no direct evidence that licensing discriminates against minority and disadvantaged groups, Hogan (1979a) reported that these groups have had unusual difficulty in obtaining appropriate credentials. The reliance of licensing laws on academic credentials—which are less frequently possessed by the poor, minorities, women, and the elderly—has a deeply pernicious and discriminating effect, especially when evidence does not exist that these credentials are positively correlated with competence (p. 282). Collins (1979) concurred: "Since the evidence strongly shows that credentials do not provide work skills that cannot be acquired on the job, and that access to credentials is inherently biased toward particular groups the case for discrimination is easy to make" (p. 198).

In medicine, Frech (1974) documented the assertion that entry restrictions had the impact on medical schools of creating a "sellers' market" so that medical schools could begin to turn away students in large numbers. This permitted medical schools to discriminate against blacks, women, Jews, and other groups in their admission policies. The 1910 Flexner report resulted in the number of black medical schools dropping from seven to two, in halting a steady increase in the percentage of black physicians (0.9 percent in 1890 to 2.7 percent in 1920), and in causing a decline to 1.4 percent by 1969. Sorkin (1977) reported that the peak in the proportion of women enrolled in medical schools occurred in 1910. The proportion and absolute number of women physicians was greater in 1910 than in 1950. Among Jews, medical school admissions during the depression of the 1930s declined by 30 percent while total admissions only declined by 13 percent. Magaro et al. (1978) estimated that 90 percent of psychiatrists and 66 percent of clinical psychologists are male, a majority are married, and they are predominantly of upper-middle-class origin.

Professional monopolies are associated with the constitutionally derived police powers and are protected by statutes making unauthorized practice a crime, indicating the seriousness with which these matters are considered. Such strong measures point out the implicit freedom-of-choice issues that emerge when people are not allowed to consult their own desired practitioners. Arguing that the U.S. Constitution should provide for medical as well as religious freedom, Benjamin Rush, first surgeon general of the army and signer of the Declaration of Independence, is reported to have said: "To restrict the act of healing to one class of men, and deny equal privileges to others will constitute the Bastille of medical science. All such laws are un-American and despotic" (Inglis, 1964, p. 5). More recently, Thomas Szasz (1977) found it "astonishing—and wonderfully revealing—how people defend the freedom of the press while they do not defend nearly so much, or not at all, freedom of education or freedom of medicine" (p. 160). Szasz countered the "society knows best" theory, believing in the need to preserve dissent.

After all, authorities never object to people agreeing with them. But they get unhappy and often quite nasty when people disagree with them. So it's disagreement that must be nurtured and protected. . . . I think we should think of it more as the right to disagree and reject authority—religious authority, educational authority, medical authority—and of course the right to take one's chances with one's own judgment and decision. [p. 162]

Freedom of choice for the consumer is more than just a theoretical postulate as questions are raised about the inability of traditional medicine to be effective in the area of chronic illness, an increasing proportion of medical practice; the inability of professionals to offer service demonstrably superior (in outcome measures) to that offered by unorthodox practitioners and self-help groups; and the difficulty an increasingly bureaucratized and impersonal professional establishment has in offering quality and caring services (Carlson, 1975).

Private Clubs

Third, [licensing] may incorporate the ethics, standards and particular interests of private associations into administrative regulations and thus give the status of public law to essentially private rules. This would result in a virtual delegation of regulatory powers to the regulated groups themselves. [Council, 1952, p. 4]

George Stigler (1971) introduced his much-quoted paper "The Theory of Economic Regulation" with the assumption that "as a rule, regulation is acquired by the industry and is designed and operated primarily for its benefit" (p. 3). He discounted two widely held alternative views. One he labeled as idealistic. Regulation is directed at the public interest and if there is injury to the public, the injury is unfortunate but it occurs in the service of a greater social goal. The second he labeled as nonrationalistic. Politics is considered an imponderable mixture of forces resulting in acts of both great virtue and vulgar veniality.

As has been noted earlier, there are few cases where regulations have been thrust on an unwilling occupation. In most instances, licensure has been sought by the regulated occupation or profession, with professional associations active in writing licensing statutes and developing administrative rules and regulations. In the case where the regulated profession plays a dominant role in the decision making of the licensing board and supports the vested interests of the occupation, it is considered "captured" by the occupation. Board members may be selected from among nominations made by the professional association, and the board may be constituted exclusively of members of the regulated profession (Cohen, 1975, pp. 124-25). The "capture" is the direct result of the ability highly concentrated, special-interest groups have to influence legislation in contrast to a widely dispersed public where a general interest provides no rallying point for concerted action.

According to Krause (1977), regulation is more important to regulated groups than to consumers. This results in differences in the degree of political organization, in the resources available and the ability to marshal special expertise, and in the co-optation and the opportunism involved in personnel changing jobs from regulatory agencies to the industries they regulate. According to a 1971 report concerning the health field, most state boards were composed of persons who directly represented the regulated groups; few boards included public representatives; approximately half of these boards required that *all* board members be licensed by the boards they serve; and faculty members in institutions training practitioners in the occupation were rarely included (Dept. of HEW, 1971).

The vested interests of professionals have led licensing boards to ignore national manpower shortages, the insufficiency of opportunity for members of minority groups, the often unnecessary length and cost of training, the problem of mobility across state lines, and the poor practice of colleagues who are out of date (Roemer, 1974; Shimberg et al. 1973). The exclusive club mentality operates to ignore the underserved—the poor, the aged, and the minorities. Though professionals are sometimes influenced by those outside their ranks, the rule is social distance from outsiders and others in lower status occupations. Such consequences are made necessary in the service of maintaining political control over the system of social stratification (gate keeping, career channels, and work definitions) that eases the way for an elite class of persons to enter into what Collins (1979) called a "status group."

Status groups are formed on the basis of common and distinctive experiences, interests and resources. Status communities may derive both from occupational and territorial (ethnic) situations: class-based status groups derive from occupational experiences, common interests in struggles for power and wealth, and differential resources for life style. . . . [T]he interests of the members in wealth, power, and prestige motivate them to institute strong collective controls over insiders and to seek monopolistic sanctions against outsiders and their resources [and] . . . enable them to organize an occupational community with strong controls and defenses. [pp. 134-35]

Innovation Restraints

Fourth, by defining the limits of particular professions and trades to include only certain existing practices and to exclude others [licensing] may inhibit the development of new techniques and skills necessary to the health, safety and welfare of the people. [Council, 1952, p. 4]

The very act of defining the scope of practice and the type of academic credentials deemed acceptable (both necessary for a licensing law) restrains innovation. According to Rogers (1973), the first and inevitable effect of setting up criteria for certification "is to freeze the profession in a past image"(p. 382).It has this effect on professional practice and on educational preparation. The passage of a practice act increases the likelihood of malpractice law suits. Carlson (1970) uses a common medical circumstance to explain that having either an unlicensed aide perform an act that requires a license to perform or having a licensed aide perform an act not included in the aide's license may constitute a presumption of negligence.

Such a presumption, although not conclusive, makes it more likely that a finding of negligence on the part of the health assistant will result—because the presumption gives the plaintiff-patient an advantage which must be overcome by the defendant. In such a case, the presumption arises because utilization of the health practitioner in the particular instance did not conform to the legislative allocation of functions and hence presumably departed from the established standard of care. [p. 852]

It is part of the irrationality of the system of licensing that it does not matter whether the unlicensed person was more capable of performing the act than the licensed person. A major factor contributing to the problem, mentioned previously, is the artificial scarcity that creates the poor utilization of manpower. Also, given the swift pace of developments in new knowledge and technology, physicians are placed in the impossible situation of being responsible for the performance of aides who have superior knowledge and skill in activities in which the physicians themselves have no or little training. This situation tends to create a type of inertia that prolongs the use of orthodox but questionable treatments (for example, lobotomy and Wasserman test) (Office, 1978) and delays the introduction of unorthodox but useful treatments (for example, acupuncture and nutrition) (Carlson, 1975) pioneered by persons outside of the established ideological framework.

The licensure system, with its formal requirements based on credentials rather than ability, restricts the beneficial movement of persons from one related occupation to another or from one type of responsibility to another. By restricting both vertical mobility (for example, career ladders) and horizontal mobility (for example, career lattices) (Dept. of HEW, 1971), the system "locks in" individuals and thereby impedes naturally occurring change which would be stimulated if personnel were more mobile. Levin (1974) recognizes this facet of the system. "No amount of interprofessional rhetoric can overcome the effects of a vocationally segregated health education organization fragmented further by impenetrable elitist credentialing barriers that prevent cumulative acquisition of progressive skills and knowledge" (p. 57).

In the training of persons in the health field, the influence of the medical profession is profound due to the control physicians exercise over licensing boards and over accreditation standards both in medicine and allied health fields. Dolan (1982) found "a staggering sameness" in training health professionals (with the exception of nursing). The rule is "industry-wide socialization and training patterns" (p. 629) supported by States that mostly use the same list of accredited schools for each profession. Since accreditation prizes uniformity, the likelihood of varied brands of professional education within a profession is virtually foreclosed. Accreditation is the lever as Krause (1977) has indicated: "Since such accreditation is usually necessary for the kind of federal money needed to keep schools going, the profession has the power of life and death over innovative training programs which might threaten its interests" (p. 284). Dolan (1982) concluded, "The ability of a consumer to go to another professional whose views are more compatible with their own is limited by the occupational licensure laws and other closed arrangements" (p. 630). The consequence, according to Havighurst (1980), followed the form of a particular ideology: "the medical schools, under substantial central control, have propagated . . . [their] strong emphasis on specialization and high-cost acute care, their inattention to cost effectiveness and efficiency, and their devaluation of primary and preventative care" (pp. 103-4). Perhaps the least visible but most profound restraint licensing has on innovation involves its emphasis on training as opposed to education. The rapid pace of change evident in these times requires more than anything else "education for uncertainty." Referring to the field of community psychology, Rappaport (1978) pleads for the education rather than the mere training of community psychologists. He distinguishes between training and education as follows:

Training implies that I have a set of very specific skills, for very specific problems, and it implies that given proper instruction these are transferable and will lead to precise performance and predictable outcomes. It suggests a technology (and of course the related tendency to obsolescence).

Education, on the other hand, is a matter of being informed about the current state of knowledge, whatever it is, and knowing how to stay informed. It implies that what is transferable, given proper instruction, are not specific skills so much as non-specific competencies. Education enables one to think about a variety of problems in a variety of ways. Training suggests professionals, specializing and licensed. Education suggests inquiry, adaptability, and flexibility, including cross disciplinary fertilization, which is difficult to license. [p. 3]

Danish and Smyer (1981) believed that an unanticipated consequence licensing has had on graduate education in psychology was to lead the field in a regressive direction. At such time as the greater specificity, necessary for accreditation and licensing, was commonly included in graduate education, it would be more difficult to change these curriculums as societal needs and problems change. This was seen as hindering the type of diverse program development and academic freedom so necessary for the education of flexible professionals. Further, Danish and Smyer saw licensing (stimulated by the prospect of national health insurance and third-party payments) as shifting the emphasis toward reimbursable individual treatment and clinical remediation strategies and away from recently developed and more broadly based preventative strategies pursued in concert with other professionals, paraprofessionals, and self-help groups. Of course, the strategies pursued by professionals would, in turn, influence the direction and scope of graduate education.

Arbitrary Action

Fifth, [licensing agencies] may take arbitrary and unreasonable action in revoking the right of persons to practice the occupations of their choice. [Council, 1952, p. 4]

As the result of bureaucratic organization and "rational" entry requirements, licensing tends to support major inroads on the right to work and to support policies of social selection that favor particular groups in the population. Also, bureaucracy is made necessary by licensing so as to manage the rationalized requirements of the enabling statute. Rules and rule makers have great difficulty in coping with ambiguity and diversity according to Rogers (1973).

Bureaucratic rules become a substitute for sound judgment. A person is disqualified because he has 150 hours of supervised therapy, while another is approved because he has the required 200. No attention is given to the effectiveness of either therapist, or the quality of his work, or even the quality of the supervision he received. Or another person is disqualified because his excellent psychological thesis was done in a graduate department that is not labeled psychology. [p. 382]

Complex rules and the slow-moving nature of the bureaucratic process "frustrate the consumer's ability to know what is happening and delays decision-making that might be in his interest until the action is effectively too late" (Krause, 1977, p. 278).

A primary way that arbitrary action is revealed is in the assessment of initial competence. The method by which licensing agencies assess initial competence is to evaluate candidates' characteristics and abilities. Four types of qualifications are examined: (1) personal characteristics such as age, citizenship, and residency in the jurisdiction; (2) educational credentials; (3) work experience such as internships or supervised practice; and (4) results of written and oral examinations. How to define and evaluate competency are, of course, controversial issues to begin with. Licensing agencies implement competency measures on the basis of what can be measured easily, despite the lack of empirical validation. Consider Pottinger's (1977) report that the sheer amount of knowledge of a content area "is generally unrelated to superior performance in an occupation . . . [or] even to minimally acceptable performance" (p. 8); yet knowledge of content is predominantly what is measured in the multiple-choice format of written licensing exams. Similarly, such requirements in psychology licensing laws as citizenship (sixteen states), local residence (ten states), and "good moral character" (forty-five states) have little relevance if one is estimating competence.

The following discussion uses material drawn from the field of psychology. Hogan (1979a) found work experience to be an excellent predictor of psychotherapeutic competence. Parloff (1979), on the other hand, found that though the "therapist's experience is related to the quality of the relationship . . . evidence regarding its association with outcome is far less clear" (p. 300). Knowing that more experienced psychotherapists are more competent than less experienced psychotherapists is not a sufficient guideline for licensing, yet numbers of years experience are what one finds in psychology licensing statutes (Hogan, 1979b).

Similarly, academic credentials are universally required, yet training does not predict psychotherapeutic competence (Parloff, 1979; Hogan, 1979a), nor are grades or degrees found to be related to professional accomplishment (Collins, 1979). The comparable psychotherapeutic effectiveness often reported for paraprofessionals, lay persons, and professionals raises a great deal of doubt about the importance of theoretical and technical knowledge (Hogan, 1979a; Parloff, 1979). With regard to diagnostic activity, Hogan (1979a) reported the serious reliability and validity problems involved in diagnostic activity. He indicated that for making gross distinctions (differentiating those who are mentally ill from those who are not) some paraprofessionals and patients are superior to professionals.

The irrelevance of entry requirements holds from one licensed occupation to another. They may be considered arbitrary since, to use Hogan's (1979a) general assessment, "There is no evidence that licensing requirements measure significant factors" (p. 255). One explanation is that the assessment techniques used in licensing occupations may have more to do with social selection than with competence. Collins (1979) discussed this process as a gate-keeping function—a means by which a dominant class controls the distribution of society's resources by maintaining a system of social stratification. He corroborates Benham's (1980) statement that a major purpose of licensing is to provide "career insurance" by describing the modern sinecure: "one invests in educational credentials, which in turn . . . are used to purchase a job protected from various aspects of labor market competition" (p. 57). The purchase of the sinecure is made available to those groups in the population who are most adept at gaining educational credentials and surviving bureaucratic mazes and it is protected by those who have a vested interest in maintaining the sinecure—the representatives of the licensed occupations. Hogan's (1979a) finding that certain groups are underrepresented in the professions provides support for the social selection hypothesis. He argued:

If academic credentials are required for entry into a profession, and if these credentials are not valid or reliable measures of competence, and if minorities, women, the poor and the aged have greater-than-normal difficulty in obtaining these credentials, then it is reasonable to assume that discrimination has taken place (whether intentional or not). [p. 281]

Interviewed in the American Psychological Association *Monitor* (Investigating, 1978) Paul Pottinger is quoted as follows:

The whole rationale for demanding scientific knowledge is strictly an arbitrary, exclusionary device. . . . If "scientificness" did not exclude a lot of people, another means would be found—practicums, publishing. They'd find something to say:"—If you haven't done this, well, you shouldn't be in the club. . . . We've got to narrow down the field, we've got to preserve the economic status of the profession. We have to be recognized as differentiated from others so our economic power and status base is preserved"—then comes all the rationale. [p. 8]

Pottinger (1980b) offered an explanation for how this works presently, based on the politics of the marketplace. If an increasing proportion of a market is financed by government, as is the case in allied health care services, professions cannot compete, in the way predicted by classical economic theory, by providing quality service at a fair price. In this situation, artificial credentials—academic degrees, licensing, and status— have value in the marketplace. Performance, outcome, and demonstrated competence do not have value partly because these are so difficult to measure. Artificial credentials are based on measures of knowledge retention which appear to make sense to the public and which are used in licensing examinations. These examinations are biased in favor of those who have followed prescribed training routes, successfully discriminating the educated from the uneducated. By doing so, the system requiring formal education is made convincing and successfully blocks alternative career entry paths for those workers who may have gained competency through apprenticeship training. Military training is an example of an alternate career entry path in the allied health care area. For persons so trained, examinations based on performance competency rather than knowledge proficiency would permit alternative entry and make unnecessary the formal education that is presently a political necessity.

These practices restrict freedom of occupational choice and even the right to work. Gellhorn (1976) believed this right, "one of the man's most precious liberties" (p. 11), had been badly eroded. In this regard, Greene (1969) indicated that "during the past quarter century [occupational licensing] laws have doubled the number of professions, skilled trades, and even semi-skilled jobs a worker cannot enter until he has demonstrated his competence and integrity to the satisfaction of a Federal, State or municipal licensing authority" (p. 2).

Hogan (1979a) estimated that occupational licensing legislation affected from one-fifth to one-third of the work force in 1976. This issue cuts rather deeply and poses a serious responsibility to licensing authorities for, according to Mackin (1976),

having power over a person's subsistence amounts to having power over a person's will. Occupational licensing can contract people's subsistence by denying them the opportunity to practice an occupation. We must review that control to insure that the license does not wrongfully control a person's will. [p. 511]

Lack of Accountability

Sixth, in many cases in which the boards control fees and funds, they may collect fees and disburse funds without adequate accounting to the legislature or the people. [Council, 1952, p. 4]

The problem of poor accounting practice is secondary to the relative absence of accountability to the public for the mission for which occupational licensing was chartered. The poor record of public accountability centers on the failure of the licensing system to protect the public. This system essentially relies on self-policing by regulated professionals through offices of the licensing agency and is based on acceptance of the professions' ethical standards.

Licensing does not seem to be effective in preventing incompetent practice nor is there much interest in disciplining incompetent practitioners. Derbyshire (1969), a former president of the Federation of State Medical Boards, estimated that 5 percent of America's physicians are unfit to practice. Makofsky (1977) estimated that approximately 30,000 Americans die each year from faulty prescriptions and ten times that number encounter severe side effects from drugs that were prescribed mistakenly. He reports on physician corruption involving Medicaid.

The following practices were disclosed: ping-ponging (sending patients from one doctor to another for unnecessary examinations and shots, the fees being charged to Medicare and Medicaid); unnecessary medication; unqualified practice; no services; and first-claim visits (doctors are allowed to charge higher fees for first visits). The Stein committee estimated that over $300 million per year has been paid to doctors for these fraudulent claims. [p. 28]

The publication *ProForum* quoted a former Pennsylvania commissioner of insurance as estimating that 15 percent of America's dentists are either incompetent or dishonest and that dentists extract six million teeth a year that could be saved through other treatment (On the Dental Front, 1979).

Ehrenreich (1978) described the course of the dawning awareness that

modern medicine was both physically and socially *harmful*. The dangers of supposedly safe medications had been publicized in the early 1960s in cases such as the Thalidomide tragedy. But it was the feminists' exposure of the dangers of oral contraceptives in the late sixties that made this a continuing concern to a mass audience. Soon information was accumulating on the prevalence of unnecessary (and often risky) surgery, on doctors' overreadiness to prescribe inappropriate or dangerous drugs, on overuse of dangerous diagnostic procedures, and more. [p. 14]

The promise of licensing proponents has been that the public can rely on licensed and autonomous professionals to protect them from harm and fraud. Licensing agencies have not only not been able to do that, they appear uninterested in doing it. Daniels (1973) concluded:

There is really no reason to accept the contention that professional autonomy best meets the requirements for maintaining standards of professional service. For whatever the rhetoric of professionalism, all the evidence seems to indicate that autonomy does not encourage the development of practical or workable systems of control. [p. 54]

The licensing agencies have responsibility for determining initial competence and for monitoring and maintaining competence; yet, according to Derbyshire, in 1969, thirty-eight states did not specify professional incompetence in their medical licensing acts as a reason for disciplinary action. For the most part, board staffs were inadequate to carry on investigations (Cohen, 1973). Cohen and Miike (1974) found that "boards did not address the broader question of systematically maintaining competence for all individuals licensed, but dealt instead, with those cases in which formal disciplinary action was indicated. Even this limited role has proven generally ineffective" (p. 267). They cited as reasons for the ineffectiveness reluctance to act against a fellow practitioner, fear of lawsuits, confusion in function since boards are both rule makers and adjudicators, and ambiguous statutory provisions. Krause (1977) found that recommendations for ways of countering these criticisms, particularly by increasing board staff to step up surveillance of professions and to conduct examinations have rarely been implemented. He concluded "the most striking finding of all studies is the near total avoidance of any policing of peers by the licensing board members even in cases of extreme malfeasance" (p. 284).

In this chapter the argument over professional licensing has been detailed. In succeeding chapters the underlying dimensions are explored and alternatives considered.

3

WHY NOW?
THE ERUPTION
OF AN ISSUE

Licensing is no longer an esoteric issue. It has become a public policy concern as questions of public accountability, cost control, discrimination, occupational recognition and competition, and public dissatisfaction have surfaced regarding the professions. Licensing is central in these matters, as Shimberg (1977) has indicated.

A confrontation is developing between the professions and the public over the matter of professional regulation. At issue are two clearly related questions: What is the purpose of licensing? And to whom do licensing boards owe their primary allegiance—to the public or to the professional groups they regulate? There is a growing feeling among the public that the purpose of licensing has been subverted. Although licensing laws were passed initially with the promise that they would provide assurance of high quality service and protect the public from incompetent practitioners, it is now alleged that the powers entrusted to licensing boards are often used to promote the interests of the licensed group at the expense of the public. [p. 154]

Licensing has long been considered the unquestioned right of certain occupations. As the result of changes occurring in the last two decades, licensing has become a public policy issue, revealing its importance and exposing its assumptions. In 1971, a Department of Health, Education, and Welfare report indicated that:

Only a few years ago, issues such as licensing, certification, and accreditation were generally thought to be the concern of only the professional individuals and organizations that were affected by them. The public-policy aspects of these issues were not often perceived by decision-makers, long accustomed to guild traditions that have characterized attitudes in this area. Today, these matters are not immune from public criticism; and the responsibility of both public and private leadership is to fuse health manpower credentialing with the public interest. [pp. 1-2]

Pottinger (1979a) described licensing as an issue that had come of age, noting that scholars began to seek larger audiences for their work on licensing. Licensing is tied up in important public policy questions with profound political, social, and economic implications.

Several forces coalesced to change licensing from a private to a public issue. An explosion of knowledge from the physical sciences led to a bio-medical engineering revolution in health care and a proliferation of new technology, techniques, and allied health specializations. New knowledge and theory in the social and behavioral sciences—led by Albert Bandura, Eric Berne, Albert Ellis, Kurt Lewin, Abraham Maslow, Fritz Perls, Carl Rogers, B. F. Skinner, and others—stimulated a variety of new techniques and specializations, leading to a revolution in awareness and interventions in the helping and mental health professions. Psychotherapy was trans-formed in its scope from a remedial, deficiency-oriented treatment into an opportunity for new learning, growth, and self-actualization. The health and helping fields have followed somewhat different scenarios, but both have been led to pursue licensing as a means to solve their problems of occupational identity. As a result there has been increasing pressure on state legislatures to credential occupations, exposing licensing to public view.

THE HEALTH OCCUPATIONS SCENARIO

The proliferation of new technology and technique such as the artificial kidney, high voltage X-ray therapy, and ultrasonic diagnostic techniques (National Advisory, 1967) led to increased specialization in the health care field. New occupations developed (for example, inhalation therapist, nu-clear medical technologist, physician's assistant) and older occupations developed new forms (for example, nurse practitioner). While the number of persons working in the older professions (for example, pharmacists, dentists, nurses, physicians) doubled between 1950 and 1967, the persons working in the allied health occupations (for example, medical technologist, optician, physical therapist, dietitian) tripled (Pennell and Hoover, 1970). Another report on the period from 1950 to 1965 showed an increase in the numbers of traditional professionals ranging from 15 percent for dentists and 17 percent for pharmacists to 33 percent for physicians and 60 percent for professional nurses. Comparisons with allied health occupations range from 116 percent for dental hygienists and 126 percent for radiologic technicians, to 183 percent for clinical laboratory personnel (National Advisory, 1967). In total, the number of persons employed in the health services rose from 1.7 million (or 2.96 percent of the employed work force) in 1950 to 4.3 million (5.6 percent) in 1970 (Knowles, 1977). The desire of allied health workers for increased recognition and income led them to follow the professionalizing scenario, originally charted by the older professions, by calling for validation through state licensing. As a result, the number of health occupations licensed in every state doubled in the last quarter of a century from eight (Council, 1952) to sixteen in 1977 (Dept. of HEW, 1979). The number of health occupations subject to licensing rose from twenty in 1952 to thirty-five in 1977 (table 3.1). An epidemic of statutory provisions was reported by Greene (1969). The provisions numbered 2,800, up 1,600 in seventeen years.

TABLE 3.1 Thirty-five Health Professions and Occupations Subject to Licensing in 1977, according to Number of Jurisdictions (All States and the District of Columbia) by Years

Occupations	1977[1] (N=51) Jurisdictions	1974[2] (N=51) Jurisdictions	1968[3] (N=51) Jurisdictions	1952[4] (N=48)[d] States
Chiropractors	51	50	49	44
Clinical laboratory services director	19	19	13	NR
Clinical laboratory services, medical technologist	10	10	10	2
Dental hygienist	51	51	51	29
Dental laboratory technician	1	1	1	NR
Dentists	51	51	51	47
Embalmer	51	51	50[sd]	48
Environmental health engineer	51	51	NR	NR
Funeral director	44	44	44[sd]	40
Midwife (lay)[a]	24	23	23	14
Midwife (nurse)	18	7	NR	NR
Nursing home administrator	51	49	49	NR
Occupational therapist	7	1	NR	NR
Occupational therapy assistant	1	1	NR	NR
Opthalmic laboratory technician	2	2	2	NR
Optician	19	17	17	7
Optometrist	51	51	51	48
Pharmacist	51	51	51	48
Physical therapist	51	51	51	15
Physical therapy assistant	22	14	10	NR
Physician (M.D.)	51	51	51	48
Physician (D.O.)	51	51	51	48
Physician's assistant[b]	33	33	6	NR
Psychiatric aide	3	3	3	NR
Podiatrist[e]	51	51	51	48
Practical nurse	51	51	51	37
Professional nurse	51	51	51	48
Psychologist	51	47	43	4

Table 3.1—*(continued)*

Occupations	1977[1] (N=51) Jurisdictions	1974[2] (N=51) Jurisdictions	1968[3] (N=51) Jurisdictions	1952[4] (N=48)[d] States
Radiologic technologist	5	3	3	NR
Inhalation therapist	1	1	1	NR
Sanitarian	36	35	35	3
Sanitarian technician	1	1	1	NR
Social Worker[c]	12	11	7	1
Speech pathologist and audiologist	29	14	NR	NR
Veterinarian	51	51	51	48

[1]Department of Health, Education, and Welfare, *Health Resources Statistics: Health Manpower and Health Facilities*, 1976-79 edition (Washington, D.C.: U.S. Government Printing Office, 1979), pp. 473-78.

[2]Department of Health, Education and Welfare, *Health Resources Statistics: Health Manpower and Health Facilities, 1974* (Washington, D.C.: U.S. Government Printing Office, 1974), pp. 536-40.

[3]M. Y. Pennell and P. A. Stewart, *State Licensing of Health Occupations* (Washington, D.C.: U.S. Government Printing Office, 1968).

[4]Council of State Governments, *Occupational Licensing Legislation in the States* (Chicago, Ill.: Council, 1952), pp. 78-103.

[5]K. Greene, *Occupational Licensing and the Supply of Nonprofessional Manpower*, Manpower Research Monograph no. 11, U.S. Department of Labor (Washington, D.C.: U.S. Government Printing Office, 1969), p. 54.

NR   Not reported.

[a]In 11 states new licenses are no longer issued though existing ones may be renewed.

[b]Delegation of function under physician's supervision.

[c]Most other sources indicate that twenty-one states license social workers (for example, Hogan, 1979b).

[d]District of Columbia not included.

[e]Listed as "chiropodist" in Council (1952).

Unwilling to share their turf with the newer occupations, the older professions expressed concerns such as this one stated by Passarelli (1979): "uncontrolled proliferation of credentialing mechanisms is cheapening the worth of the function as a whole and may ultimately throw it into meaninglessness" (p. 118). The Department of Health, Education, and Welfare recommended a two-year state legislative moratorium on licensing new health-related occupations in 1971, which was renewed for another two years (Dept. of HEW, 1971, 1976) attempting to slow down the proliferation process. This did not stop the trend that saw thirty new laws in 1974 in the health field (Hogan, 1979a). The moratorium was often coupled with calls for the reform of licensing laws which, particularly in the health occupations, "have impeded the allocation of different functions to existing allied health personnel and discouraged the development of new types of paramedical personnel" (Carlson, 1970, p. 851). Envoking a theme we shall see repeated throughout this book, Fine (1971) attributed the resistance to what he called the myth of professionalism

which has distorted our health care system . . . [and] which shrouds the delivery of many health services in secrecy. Like a medieval guild the medical profession has arbitrarily determined that certain procedures can be performed only by a physician—not on the basis of unique skill involved, but purely on the basis of tradition. [p. 12]

THE "HELPING" OCCUPATIONS SCENARIO

At the same time, chaos was the order of the day in the realm of the helping professions—an exploding tangle of human services, alternative therapies, new institutions, and nontraditional helping occupations. There were paraprofessionals and counselors in such traditional institutions as schools, churches, prisons, recreation facilities, manpower agencies, mental health and social agencies, drug treatment centers, and hospitals as well as in "growth centers" and private practice. Community mental health centers and social welfare agencies, often supported by federal funds, employed and trained paraprofessionals to link their institutions to poor, minority, and other special populations. Universities trained agency, family, drug, and correctional counselors and mental health technicians while growth centers and associations trained and certified group facilitators, and gestalt, bio-energetics, and transactional analysis therapists, leaders, and consultants primarily for the middle classes. In the graduate departments of applied psychology, humanistic, behavioral, and cognitive theories began to replace analytic orientations. In 1975, Tennov estimated that the number of different therapeutic methods exceeded one hundred, increasing from thirty-six in 1959.

Also at the same time, psychiatry's hold on psychotherapy loosened as the focus of intervention theory shifted from deficiency to learning and growth models. Tennov (1975) commented that the insistence of psychiatrists on the M.D. degree as the basic qualification for psychotherapy

undermined the medical profession's hold over psychotherapeutic practice in the United States. It is ironic that by failing to extend their domain beyond medicine, M.D.'s allowed alternative psychotherapies to develop among nonphysicians. Thus clinical psychologists, social workers, marriage counselors, members of the clergy and educators began to practice psychotherapy. [p. 125]

A similar situation exists presently with regard to the insistence of the American Psychological Association on the Ph.D. as the basic qualification for membership in the Association and for psychological practice under state licensing laws. The rapid development of the American Mental Health

Counselors Association and the National Association of School Psychologists is believed to be benefiting from the APA's intransigence about admitting masters-level psychologists as full members. An excerpt from a recent social work text illustrates the problem that traditional helping professions have had in responding to the influx of new techniques.

> Social work technique is alive and well and expanding in all directions, into groupwork and encounter, human potential and personal effectiveness methods, the use of behavioural objectives and treatment contracts, task-centered casework, cocounseling, transactional analysis, social skills training, role-play, games, simulations, and many other areas.
>
> But these expanding prospects do not appear to have brought joy to all those who work in the helping agencies. On the contrary, the soul of social work seems to be sick, weighed down from above by a burgeoning bureaucracy and under attack from below by a radical sociology perspective which suggests that it amounts to little more than an insidious and dishonest form of social control. Caught in this dilemma, some workers have made use of the new methods in a piecemeal way in community work, groupwork, and, increasingly, in intermediate treatment schemes. Others have sought to elevate welfare rights advocacy into a new orthodoxy almost as narrow as the one it was intended to replace. And others have invested their energies in the pursuit of a professionalism that is somehow above all of these controversies. Mainstream social work has continued to plough a median furrow between using conventional methods, and engaging in those administrative activities that claim an increasing proportion of its time and energy. Meanwhile the manuals of new technique sit on the shelf, their pages largely unturned. And the people on the receiving end, the people with the problems, continue to pay for it all—literally, through their direct and indirect taxes on the one hand and, figuratively, through the receipt of a needlessly second-class service on the other. [Priestley et al., 1978, p. 3]

With the advent of private and federal health insurance providing coverage for mental health problems and with the advent of laws permitting professionals other than psychiatrists to receive third-party payments (twenty-eight states had freedom-of-choice laws in 1977 according to Dörkin [1977]), the issue was joined. Since 60 percent of the payments for physicians' services in 1975 came from third-party payers (Knowles, 1977), freedom-of-choice legislation has had profound implications for the economics of health and helping professions. These circumstances have placed new pressures on the state legislatures. Hogan (1979a) reported that

> the fact that so many professional groups are claiming psychotherapy as their territory has been a strong force that in itself has caused further licensing, since all relevant professions want to protect their right to practice. The prospect of national health insurance and the willingness of private insurance carriers to reimburse the treatment of mental illness by psychotherapeutic means has contributed to the proliferation of licensing, since reimbursement is generally predicated on whether a practitioner possesses a license. [p. 248]

Psychiatrists, unwilling to share what has been their exclusive occupational preserve, attempt to define psychotherapy as "medical psychotherapy" to fend off clinical psychologists who also have been battling them for hospital privileges. For their part, psychologists try to pass restrictive practice acts to deal with the threat to their turf from counselors. Of the fifty-one jurisdictions licensing psychologists in 1977, twenty-seven had practice restriction acts (Hogan, 1979a). Psychology had been licensed in forty-three jurisdictions in 1968 (Pennell and Stewart, 1968) and four in 1952 (Council, 1952). In 1979, sunset laws reduced that number to forty-nine. With some states considering new laws and others sunsetting theirs, the situation is unstable. At this writing social workers are licensed in twenty-one states, marriage counselors in six, and counselors in six.

Protection of the right to practice (or its converse, eliminating competitive practices) and maintaining eligibility for third-party reimbursement is the basis for infighting among the mental health professions. The Association for the Advancement of Psychology's publication, *Advance* carried this quote from the May 1978 *American Medical News*.

The gloves are off; psychiatrists are declaring war on anyone trying to move in on their territory. In the fight for professional survival, they have decided to align themselves with the rest of organized medicine . . . and push for treatment supremacy over allied health professionals practicing in the mental health field. [Special Projects, 1979, p. 7]

Psychologists applauded the outcome of the freedom-of-choice suit of the Virginia Academy of Clinical Psychologists against two Blue Cross/Blue Shield organizations and the Neuropsychiatric Society of Virginia, which permitted direct reimbursement for psychological services. Counselors watched the decision of the Veterans' Administration to exclude nonlicensed counseling psychologists and wondered about Lindenberg's (1976) statement that counseling is "either on the threshold of autonomy or on the threshold of dissolution as a separate and equal profession compatible with all of the helping professions" (p. 34). At the same time, substance abuse counselors (who hold their jobs because of their highly relevant life experiences) feared that any credentialing will exclude them by emphasizing schooling over experience.

The issue for counselors is an example of the effect of licensing on an occupation. The specific threat to counselors comes from legislation that restricts practice utilizing "psychological procedures" to psychologists—procedures, many of which counselors share with psychologists, social workers, and other helping professionals. The practice restriction does not affect professions already recognized by a licensing statute of their own (for example, social work) or specifically excluded in the psychology licensing law (for example, clergy). The effects in jurisdictions where counselors are not licensed is multiple. Restrictive legislation excludes even counselors with doctoral degrees from practicing their profession, reducing the social value of their qualifications to a level indistinguishable from those of the public at large. The right to practice counseling, both privately and in some institutional settings (for example, Veterans' Administration), is threatened. Counselors in these circumstances are not permitted to receive payments for services from insurance companies or other third-party payers. These influences affect the existence of counseling occupations, discouraging the development of new approaches and limiting the quality and breadth of services offered to the public. Many counselors have become so worried about their public credibility under these circumstances that they have responded by identifying with the more traditional professions. A "bandwagon" psychology has developed in which licensing of counselors is presented as the only alternative to restrictive legislation (Cottingham, 1975; Swanson, 1976; Sweeney and Sturdevant, 1974).

CONSUMER REACTION

New technology and increased specialization also lead to an inflation of costs and an acceleration of bureaucratization in the health care field. Increases in the costs of health services were estimated to be at twice the rate of other goods and services making up the consumer price index (Fine, 1971). As a percentage of the gross national product, costs in health rose from 5.2 percent in 1960 to 9 percent in 1978 (Office, 1978).

A more bureaucratized and impersonal health service system has developed where over 70 percent of American physicians are specialists, leaving only one primary care physician for every 4,771 people (Knowles, 1977). Freidson (1970) noted that health care began to resemble care traditionally provided for the indigent, characterized by "inflexibility and brevity in the way service is provided, lack of concern for the personal convenience and desires of the patient and a growing fragmentation of the services themselves" (p. 197). A bureaucratization of medicine has the effect, according to Mechanic (1976),

of diluting the personal responsibility of the provider, making it more likely that interests other than those of the patient will prevail. By segmenting responsibility for patient care, the medical bureaucracy relieves the physician of direct continuing responsibility. . . . [W]hen responsibility is less clear it is easier to make decisions in the name of other interests such as research, teaching, or demonstration. [pp. 54-55]

In response, a new criticism has developed, focusing on "such conditions as the inaccessibility of services, unnecessary surgery, excessive prescription of drugs, unexplained hospital bills, which are adversely affecting the health, well-being, and confidence of many individuals in America"

(Graubard, 1977, p. v). At the same time, the consumer self-care and self-help movements have gained new prominence and we have witnessed an epidemic of malpractice claims.

Fauri (1977) illustrated the dynamics of impersonal and condescending treatment as the basis of clients' present negative reaction to professionals.

Many of today's professionals are organization based. They work in organizations and depend on organizations for their income. . . . [T]he professional so employed is in a position to use his abilities in assisting the organization in its problem functions. . . . Under these conditions, the danger exists of the professional becoming task-oriented rather than person-oriented. . . . It may become necessary to treat people in an impersonal, abstract manner in order to accomplish the work at hand. Professional judgment may be involved in determining what is best for the client. . . . Add to this the complexities of bureaucratic rules and the client is put into a situation of dependency. . . . [C]ondescending attitudes are prevalent in professional conduct in the public sector. Seventy-eight percent of urban social workers responding to the survey believed a major part of their responsibility was to "teach" the poor how to live. [pp. 245-47]

Rosen et al. (1977) noted pervasive, wide-ranging criticism and hostility toward health institutions stimulated by high costs and inadequacies in the organization and delivery of health care. The emergence of consumer demands for change "emphasizes that widespread dissatisfaction with professional decision-making in the health system is part of the movement toward castigation and denigration of all social institutions" (p. 10).

Higher expectations about what medicine should be able to accomplish and prevent paralleled a shift in expectations from health being a privilege to health being everyone's right. Self-care has emerged "to promote the public health, control preventable disease, manage chronic illness and reduce iatrogenesis" (Levin et al., 1979, p. 78). Levin et al. viewed self-care as an emerging social movement with its roots in populism but finding current expression from the impetus of (1) costs of traditional health care; (2) new concepts and techniques (for example, holistic health, biofeedback, and Eastern therapies such as yoga and acupuncture; (3) ineffectiveness of many forms of professional care; (4) increased public determination to assert personal control over health services; and (5) increased visibility of self-care techniques (for example, jogging, meditation, natural foods, and self-care publications). Such books as the Boston Women's Health Book Collective's *Our Bodies, Ourselves* (1973) demystify and publicize knowledge physicians usually keep to themselves (for example, specific information about human sexuality). Similarly, treatment, training, and support groups offer an alternative to the awe of the professional, particularly in areas that are controversial or that professionals tend to ignore or about which they are ill informed (for example, rape crisis centers) (Lopata, 1976),

The self-care movement as a result constitutes a threat to the privileged economic position of professionals who fear that "its development will surely result in demystifying professional functions and may cause a rewriting of medicine's social charter" (Levin et al., 1979, p. 40). Riessman (1979) saw the desire of the American public for expanded and improved health care. He called for a redefinition of responsibility.

Medical professionals must be freed from work that falls outside their province. So, for example, while diagnosis, prescription, and monitoring are clearly professional activities, prevention and support of the chronically ill are not. This will mean severely weakening the health industry monopoly and all that it connotes—the traditional medical model, the over-utilization of doctors, hospitals, technical equipment, the third party payment system and the emphasis on treatment rather than health promotion and maintenance. [p. 8]

The self-help movement is characterized by relatively small and supportive face-to-face groups and a spate of popularly written literature which attempts to translate technical knowledge for lay audiences. Gartner and Riessman (1977) viewed the development of the self-help movement as a profound critique of professionalism.

Self-help mutual aid groups have developed, in large measure, because of the unwillingness and inability of professional organizations to deal with these and other problems and because of such organization's overly intellectualized orientation, excessive credentialism and limited reach in regard to various populations. [p. 12]

Paxton (1979) indicated that there are over one-half million different self-help groups operating in the United States. Covering almost any conceivable problem or concern, these groups include "drug abusers, Vietnam veterans, alcoholics, widows, families of prisoners, abusive parents, the handicapped and victims of nearly every major disease" (p. 7).

The mid-1970s saw an explosion in malpractice claims and costs. Cohen (1979) reported that (1) 1975 saw twice as many medical malpractice suits as 1970; (2) the ratio of claims to insured physicians of one insurance company changed from one to twenty-three in 1969 to one to ten in 1974; (3) claims in New York State doubled between 1970 and 1974; and (4) during a fourteen-month period in 1974 and 1975, one in seven physicians in Cook County, Illinois (Chicago) were being sued, with settlements averaging $8,000 more than settlements averaged in 1970. This flurry of activity was accompanied by increases in liability insurance premiums, in charges for medical care, and in activity by state legislatures to contain the problem by passing limitation of liability legislation.

Though the epidemic has passed, the disease is still with us. Cohen (1979) advised that increased litigation as a way of remedying perceived wrongs was partly the result of official misconduct in government, business, and labor unions, which has people more suspicious of authority. This suspicion was caused partly by the current emphasis on patient rights and assertiveness, partly by unreasonably high expectations of services, and partly by the prospect of "easy money." Makofsky (1977) cited the widespread problem of incompetent physicians, estimated to be 5 percent of practicing doctors, resulting in 30,000 American deaths each year. He noted that although Americans spent more money than other countries on health care, we had an infant mortality rate exceeding fourteen other nations and a male life expectancy shorter than that of 19 other countries. Table 3.2 describes the changes over a thirty-year period. Makofsky identified the commercial factors involved, indicating that a deliberately arranged shortage of physicians results in their earning a great deal of money while the American public is "forced to accept any medical care it can get on the doctors' terms" (p. 26). The anger over this squeeze play finds its expression in malpractice claims because when a wrong is done, there is no other way to take effective action (that is, medical societies and state licensing boards are reluctant to act) even though money rarely adequately compensates for poor health care.

The malpractice epidemic and the consumer, self-care, and self-help movements reflect various degrees of deep-seated resentment toward professionals' behavior. Professionals gain autonomy—the right to determine their own activity and to judge its consequences—from the licensing charter because they have convinced the public of their expertise and altruism. Public confidence in the knowledge and the ethical basis of professional service has been challenged because the expertise of the practitioners is inadequate and their claims to altruism are unfounded.

TABLE 3.2 Comparison of Selected Indicators of Health Status with Personal Health Care Expenditures between 1940 and 1970, United States

Indicator	1940	1955	Index Number	1970	Index Number
Infant mortality Rate[a]	47.0	26.4		20.0	
Change index (1940 = 100)			56		43
Male life expectancy at birth (years)	60.8	66.7		67.1	
Change index (1940 = 100)			110		110

Table 3.2—*(continued)*

Indicator	1940	1955	Index Number	1970	Index Number
Female life expectancy at birth (years)	65.2	72.8		74.8	
Change index (1940 = 100)			112		115
Male Life expectancy age forty (years)	30.0	31.7		31.9	
Change index (1940 = 100)			106		107
Female life expectancy age forty (years)	33.3	36.7		38.3	
Change index (1940 = 100)			110		115
Personal health care expenditures (billion dollars per year)	3.5	15.2		60.1	
Change Index (1940 = 100)			434		1717

Source: J. Ehrenreich, ed., *The Cultural Crisis of Modern Medicine* (New York: Monthly Review Press, 1978), p. 11.

[a]Deaths per 1,000 live births in the first year of life.

4

A SHORT HISTORY
OF LICENSING

The matter of state involvement in restricting who should serve the public is age old. The Babylonian Code of Hammurabi (about 2080 B.C.) stipulated both the fees patients were to pay for medical services and the punishments for negligent treatment. Women specifically were barred from medical practice in Greece about 300 B.C. An examining and licensing board existed for healers in Baghdad in 931 A.D.

EUROPEAN FOUNDATIONS

Roger II of Sicily in 1140 A.D. proclaimed an edict that penalized persons practicing medicine without a license. In 1225 a medical practice law of Frederick II, Holy Roman Emperor, reflected some of the elements of the protection problem which hold to this day. Its licensing provisions forbade practice without a license and included examination by a teacher of medicine. Punishment of offenders was to occur by confiscation of goods and a year in prison. Three years were to be devoted to the study of logic. After five years of academic study, the prospective practitioner was to engage in one year of practice under the direction of an experienced physician. Fees were set, free care for the poor was required, and a prohibition was levied on a physician owning an apothecary shop.

The power of the State was enlisted to gain a monopoly for favored medical practitioners by setting educational, examination, and experience requirements for providers. In setting fees, obliging a doctor to give the poor free care, and prohibiting ownership of a pharmacy, the implications of abuse of power from a conflict of interest were also recognized. This problem of conflict of interest had been recognized as early as the fourth century B.C. in the Hippocratic oath. This creed urged the Greek physician to do no harm; to adopt regimens for the benefit of patients; to reject the entreaties of those who would urge the giving of deadly drugs; to refrain from wrong doing, corruption, or seduction; to reject aid to women seeking abortions; and to keep silent about what was seen or heard.

By requiring that three years be spent in the study of logic, Frederick II's law had the effect of enhancing the medical occupation by reserving healing practice to the university-educated upper classes and making illegal the folk practitioners who served the mass of the public. Though excluding these informally educated practitioners tended to create a monopolistic advantage for a profession, Friedson (1970) hastened to point out that it was the twentieth century in the United States before physicians were able to put a strong occupational organization, university training, and state legislation together to form a functioning monopoly. Even then, there have been exceptions (for example, chiropractors).

From the earliest times distinctions were in effect that licensing later served to legitimize. Krause (1977) pointed to a pattern, dating from ancient Egypt and Greece, of a medical practice hierarchy that differentiated those who served the masses from those who served the elite. At the top of this hierarchy was temple medicine with its priests serving the aristocracy. At the next level were the community practitioners who practiced a fee-for-service medicine for those who could afford it and who served as the precursors of practitioners today. At the bottom was folk medicine practiced mostly by women. Ehrenreich and English (1973) described these practitioners:

Women have always been healers. They were pharmacists, cultivating healing herbs and exchanging the secrets of their uses. They were midwives, travelling from home to home and village to village. For centuries women were doctors without degrees, barred from books and lectures, learning from each other, and passing on experience from neighbor to neighbor and mother to daughter. They were called "wise women" by the people, witches or charlatans by the authorities. [p. 3]

Ehrenreich and English (1973) also noted the dichotomy in medical practice that emerged in thirteenth-century Europe, where "witches" practiced among the people while the ruling classes were served by university-trained physicians. Licensing laws came into vogue as the means "to prohibit all but university-trained doctors from practice" (p. 17). As a result of the requirement for university training, the official practice of healing was restricted to the upper classes, to men, and to those in the favor of the Church (which controlled the universities), most of whom were ecclesiastics (Council, 1952). Though the effectiveness of these laws was limited because of the great need for service and the inability and unwillingness of university-trained physicians to serve the masses, it is important to note this early reliance on the authority of the State to legitimize an occupation. This attempt to monopolize medical practice in situations of imbalance between need and available service was unrealistic because of the comparatively few licensed medical advisers and would eventually lead to a temporary abandonment of licensing in the nineteenth century in the United States (Kett, 1968).

The association between education and licensing was made in the early European laws. Marieskind (1980) pointed out that Frederick II in 1225 "attempted to confer by authoritative Bull licenses to graduates of his new school at Naples" (p. 118). Pope Gregory IX did the same in Toulouse in 1229, and these actions were repeated in virtually every other university then extant. The case of Jacoba Felicie de Almonia in 1322 is cited as an early example. Despite her defense on the grounds that it was appropriate for women to treat women, much testimony to the excellence of her skill, and the lack of any testimony about her incompetence, she was forced to suspend medical practice because of the law dating to 1220 that restricted such practice to members of the faculty of the University of Paris. The charge against her was "that—as a woman—she dared to cure at all" (Ehrenreich and English, 1973, p. 19). This approach was supported by Pope John XXII in 1325, though some twenty-five years later women were permitted to practice medicine. They were however, restricted to specific tasks.

This regulatory activity was an outgrowth of a thirteenth-century revival of learning, stimulated by European contact with the Arab world, which also resulted in the development of univerity-related medical schools. The preeminent place of the Church in European life had restricted the development of scientific medicine for some eight centuries and still controlled the practice of medicine—lest attention to the body distract attention from the soul.

Merchant guilds, which would later serve as models for professional associations, were developing at this same time and becoming the predominant form of economic organization. According to Gerstl and Jacobs (1976),

the guilds defined, defended and exercised the guildsmen's rights and their monopoly of skill. This was legitimized by the church as fitting into the cosmological order— work was a calling. . . . [T]he guilds became the primary *organizing* bodies of the medieval town and were self-governing. [p. 2]

Thus was fashioned at this time a tie between an occupation (a calling), its organization (a guild), and the expectation that a monopoly of practice was appropriate. According to Carman (1958) both university and guild tied education to licensing, serving to set in motion the future ties between the State and the professions.

The medieval universities both trained and licensed. In reality, a degree was a certificate of competence which in the cases of law and medicine usually conveyed certain exclusive rights of practice to its holder. Similarly, the guilds which evolved into

professional bodies often gave training and always attempted to give exclusive rights
of practice to their members. [p. 269]

By the sixteenth century as the universities became more secularized, the
university-trained professionals no longer were compelled to take religious
orders. Emerging from the grip of the Church, the associations of physicians
became similar to craft guilds. These, however, were not destroyed by the
impact of commercialism, centralized governments, and laissez-faire economics, as the craft guilds and the feudal system were to be (Council, 1952).
As occupations, professions were a special case, first in serving the social
elite and later in being populated by an elite. Professions, like land, broke
the direct connection between work and income for the English gentleman,
permitting him to make a considerable sum of money without engaging in a
"despised" trade. Gerstl and Jacobs (1976) concluded, "One could carry on
commerce by sleight of hand while donning the vestments of professional
altruism" (p. 3). In 1422 the English parliament required university graduation for all physicians. In 1511 Henry VIII established the College of
Physicians and Surgeons, giving it and the archbishop of Canterbury the
power to license physicians. Though the traditional connection between
licensing, the university, and the Church was maintained, the College of
Physicians and Surgeons introduced representatives of the practitioners to
participate in the licensing process. This pattern of relationship between
providers, the State, education, and the Church was brought by the early
settlers to the American colonies. Despite the fact that in 1523 the English
parliament permitted nonclergy to practice medicine for the first time,
Collins (1979) pointed out that the tradition of clergy dominance of
medicine persisted in the early colonies. Collins revealed that this mix of
church, university, and guild organization of medical providers was but a
manifestation of

a long tradition, not only of making oneself culturally acceptable to the dignified
upper class, but also of taking a priestly role toward clients. During the long
majority of medical history when no practical cures existed, ritual manipulation and
its attendant secrecy and mystification were the *sine qua non* of the occupation's
existence. Western medicine branched off from the religious studies of the medieval
university. . . . Pursuing the medical tradition back to antiquity, we find . . . the
tradition of the shaman, a role from which medicine, divination, and priestcraft all
developed. Physicians thus have an unbroken tradition of emphasizing ritual
exclusion for the purposes of occupational impressiveness. [p. 173]

EARLY AMERICAN REGULATION

The transplanting of this European tradition into the American colonies
involved several problems of transition. At first the need was great and the
number of university-educated medical practitioners was small. An appren-

ticeship tradition developed that dominated medical practice well past the time of the opening of the first medical school in the 1760s. The guild system was declining in England during the period of early immigration and craft labor was scarce in the colonies; therefore, the guild system never took root in America. This circumstance permitted the development of a commercial class of entrepreneurs. One similarity was that university training was denied to all but the wealthy since it required study in England or Europe.

The first physician-licensing statutes—Virginia in 1639, Massachusetts in 1649, and New York in 1665—were motivated more by the complaints of excessive charges than by the need to restrict practice. It was the middle of the eighteenth century, more than 100 years after the early settlers arrived, before practice restrictions were established. In 1729 the first bar association was formed in New York City. The 1760s saw the appearance of local and colony medical societies (New Jersey in 1766) and medical schools (Columbia in 1767). Shortly thereafter, in 1772, the first comprehensive medical practice act was passed by New Jersey. By 1800 thirteen of the sixteen states had given the authority to examine and license to the state medical societies. The existence of a two-tiered hierarchy of regular medical practice that included the university educated as well as the apprentice trained was recognized by the legislators, though Shryock (1967) observed that legislators were more impressed with the former group. Three parallels with the present day were evident at the turn of the nineteenth century. First, licensing was associated with the interests of the dominant elite—the Church and aristocracy in Europe and the commercial class in America (Reiff, 1974). Second, sanctioning power was given to guildlike professional organizations as the means by which these interests were to be maintained. Third, admission to the guild maintained the profession's upper-class identification by requiring, where it could, and otherwise preferring, a period of prolonged university training unavailable to the lower classes. Differing patterns existed, however, with regard to whether educational institutions, professional organizations, or the states carried the actual authority to license. As of 1803 the Harvard degree or a license granted by the medical society qualified a person to practice medicine in Massachusetts. In Connecticut, on the other hand, Yale University gave the degrees and the Connecticut Medical Society granted the licenses. The proliferation of proprietary medical schools beginning early in the nineteenth century worked to weaken the authority of the medical schools, eventually ending their direct involvement in licensing physicians. Hogan (1979a) pointed out, however, that after the deregulation in the second quarter of the nineteenth century, medical school diplomas were the only available symbol of "competence." This worked to improve the status of medical school graduates in comparison to apprenticeship doctors and established such training as the norm for preparation. Tabachnik (1976) reported that in 1800 there were four medical schools in the country, thirty in 1840, and seventy-seven in 1876.

The level of competency of the licensed practitioner was a grave question. Training programs in medical schools varied in length from a few months to two years. Most medical schools had no clinical facilities. There was little in the way of medical sciences except "heroic" measures (for example, massive bleeding, huge doses of laxatives). This was the state of so-called regular licensed medical practice at the turn of the nineteenth century. There remained unlicensed folk practitioners who filled for the masses of people the void left by the scarcity, expense, social distance, and inadequacies of the regulars. Ehrenreich and English (1973) compared them: "The lay practitioners were undoubtedly safer and more effective than the 'regulars.' They preferred mild herbal medications, dietary changes and hand-holding to heroic interventions. Maybe they didn't know any more than the 'regulars,' but at least they were less likely to do the patient harm" (p. 24).

DEREGULATION

The second quarter of the nineteenth century brought about substantial changes in the United States. In response to the egalitarian sentiment of the times, there was a wholesale deregulation of the professions of law and medicine. By the time of the Civil War, "no effective state licensing system was in operation" (Council, 1952, p. 19). The popular rhetoric explaining this eventuality has a modern sound. It included complaints that the professions (1) made things so complicated that intelligent persons who ordinarily could be expected to take responsibility for themselves could not argue in a court of law or obtain the information needed to properly take care of their health, (2) were monopolies in restraint of trade, (3) maintained a subordinating class system that hoarded privileges and blocked the entry of the lower classes, and (4) retarded developments and blocked talent in nonorthodox realms of practice (Tabachnik, 1976). More fundamentally, the demands of a growing population and an expanding frontier ushered in a wave of democracy and individualism (Council, 1952) and a popular health movement (Ehrenreich and English, 1973) that upset the machinery by which professional practice was controlled. The professions then became more socially inclusive as the society became more egalitarian.

Collins's (1979) analysis centered on the beginnings of a national corporate economy developing during this period which enhanced the survival of both small-scale local businesses and professions. They were functions "of a naturally wealthy, geographically far-flung, politically decentralized society" (p. 79). An early expression was the radical populism of the Jacksonian era which derided professional knowledge and intellectual arrogance, hoping thereby to create a more open society. In medicine this represented a radical assault on the assumptions and privileges of the "regulars." Caring for oneself was honored while "regulars" were attacked as parasites "who survived only because of the upper class' 'lurid taste' for calomel [a mercury-based laxative] and bleeding" (Ehrenreich and English, 1973, p. 25). Universities were criticized as places to learn to identify with the upper classes and to look down on others. New medical philosophies, particularly eclecticism, Grahamism, and homeopathy, set up their own medical schools and were so successful they made the old "regulars" appear to be just another medical sect.

The legal profession fared no better. The privileged position of lawyers together with the perquisites of wealth and honor were regarded widely with jealousy and resentment. The long period of apprenticeship was attacked and led to the virtual elimination of an admission requirement to practice law between 1830 and 1850. In some states good moral character and eligibility to vote were the only requirements, while others retained an examination by the admitting court. The populist ideal that every intelligent man could be his own lawyer was as close to being realized as it ever would be in modern society.

The experience with deprofessionalization in the second quarter of the nineteenth century is viewed differently in different quarters. Tabachnik (1976) reported that in America deprofessionalization stimulated the growth of medical schools, increased the number of doctors, raised average standards, and was not as bad as the leaders of American medicine at that time expected it to be. Shryock (1967), on the other hand, treats it as a calamity—a time of rampant quackery and deterioration in the quality of practice. It is never clear in his analysis if quality is related to competence or to the social class and educational background of the physician.

THE BEGINNING OF MODERN LICENSING

In the latter half of the nineteenth century a variety of factors coalesced into a reversal of the deregulating trend. According to Haskell (1977) there was an inclination among the mass of the public that "threatened to withhold deference from all men, all traditions, and even the highest values" (p. 65) because the world was so uncertain (first post-Jacksonian and then post-Darwinian). The professionalizing trend was a means by which authority could be established that would counter the uncertainty. He points to the social origins of doubts that would result in new ways of escaping uncertainty.

The social sciences rose to cultural dominance at a time of rampant doubt and uncertainty among the better educated members of western society. The late nineteenth century is commonly understood to be a period of spiritual crisis when the Christian cosmology weakened by the rude shock of Darwin's evolutionary theory first lost its grip on substantial parts of the intellectual class. But the exhaustion of faith and the growing popularity of naturalists and uniformitarian views may themselves have been induced by subtle changes in the patterns of social experience. Certainly the inability of sensitive minds to attribute causation unambiguously in everyday affairs must have compounded the crisis of confident belief, even if the belief has independent origins. [pp. 44-45]

One result was to form professional societies, referred to as "communities of the competent," which had institutional frameworks, to "identify individual competence, cultivate it, and confer authority upon the individuals who possessed it" (Haskell, 1977, p. 65). The professional society served to insulate scientists against public opinion—those who were least competent to judge them—while bringing them in close competitive exposure to each other—those who were most competent to judge them—thus securing a distant and uncluttered avenue of influence over the public. To gain entrance to this elite group, scientists could no longer be ordinary citizens. Their authority in the eyes of the public would be enhanced when they took their places in a group where membership was based on occupational competence, presuming, of course, a favorable judgment by their occupational peers.

The first association having these characteristics was formed by geologists in 1840 and expanded in 1847 to become the American Association for the Advancement of Science. Then other science-related professions followed. The physicians organized in 1847, followed by the pharmacists and the civil engineers in 1852, the architects in 1857, the dentists in 1859, and the veterinarians in 1863. The American Bar Association was not to form, however, until 1877. These associations concerned themselves with gaining dominance over their fields using the tactics of licensing and accreditation of training programs. The physicians and other health occupations had to deal with the increasingly divided sectarian and lay practitioners. All professionals had to disguise their entrepreneurial nature so as not to be "regarded as mere businessmen but as members of a profession" (Carman, 1958, p. 278).

With the growing power of the associations and their reservation of the determination of competency, the so-called scientific professions were ready to make their final and ultimately successful assault to gain monopolistic power by tying in the interests of the State with the interests of the professions. The linking of competency with licensing by demanding regulations to end quackery, supposedly protecting the public, was a brilliant and ultimately winning argument. The previous low status of the professions during the period of deregulation was associated in the rhetoric, with the practice of ignorant, unprincipled persons who did not have suitable preparation for serving the public. These ideas gained the stature of a reform movement based on the twin virtues of reason and science. Collins (1979) also noted that the reform movement at the turn of the twentieth century mobilized the Anglo-Protestant middle class to react to the massive immigration of persons from Europe. Gerstl and Jacobs (1976) discussed the motivating force behind licensing to include the vulnerability felt by professionals who were less able in these tempestuous times to use the class system to maintain a privileged status for the university educated. Thus they turned toward government to secure public confidence and a monopoly of skill. Ehrenreich and English (1973) described the development of a women's health movement at this time which, in an effort to achieve respectability, disassociated itself from the popular health movement. Female medical leaders were co-opted into supporting a sexist regular medical profession. It is no small wonder that when this reform movement was later successful, medicine would be described as a "white, male, middle class occupation" (Ehrenreich and English, 1973, p. 33).

The first modern medical practice act was passed in Texas in 1873, with California following in 1875. By 1905 thirty-nine states licensed physicians (Council, 1952). Nurses formed a national association in 1896, had New York and Virginia adopt statutes licensing nurses in 1903, and by 1926 had forty states licensing nurses.

At this same time the Supreme Court was pursuing a doctrine based on the equal protection clause of the Fourteenth Amendment, the substantive guarantee of due process, which required legislation to have a rational relationship to some legitimate end of government. Without such relationship, the law was seen to unconstitutionally deprive those concerned of their liberty. The doctrine was named "substantive due process" and was the means by which the Court enforced its ideas about the desirability of a free-market economic system. It was a doctrine that supported economic expansion and that would support occupational freedom and resist licensure. This was not to be the case as the Court, in the 1888 case of *Dent* v. *West Virginia*, made an exception for medical licensure under the more ancient doctrine of the State's police powers. A state law purporting to protect the health, welfare, or safety of citizens was justified as having a rational relationship to the legitimate end of government, under the police-power banner. Though for fifty years the Court would examine police power exceptions under the substantive doctrine, *Dent* v. *West Virginia* opened the floodgates to occupational licensure. Court action interfering with state police powers has been rare, but it has barred attempts to force disclosure of political affiliation and to restrict advertising, both under the rubric of the First Amendment to the Constitution. The failure to conduct a fair hearing has been considered a violation of the due process clause of the Fourteenth Amendment.

The fight for control over training programs began a bit later. The first modern medical school was founded at Johns Hopkins in 1893 by scientific reformers using the germ theory as a rational basis for disease prevention and treatment. Organized philanthropy based on fortunes earned in oil and coal was caught up in this reformist spirit and became involved in the creation of a "truly" scientific medical profession. The AMA's Council on Medical Education, initially formed in 1904, had difficulty with the medical schools in its accreditation project. At the behest of the Council in 1910, Abraham Flexner of the Carnegie Corporation published a report on medical education that became the first effective accreditation effort backed as it was by the promise of foundation financial support. Flexner used the Johns Hopkins Medical School as a model and recommended that those not conforming be shut down. The AMA was to gain effective control over medical training. Within five years, 40 percent of the medical schools were closed, and twenty years later only one unapproved school still survived.

Several patterns, developed during the twentieth century experience with licensing, were elaborations of patterns already set. These included a steady increase in the number of licensed occupations, an increased centralization in the control of licensing, a switching from title-restricting laws to practice-restricting laws, and an increased evidence of greater exclusiveness in eligibility standards.

Traditionally, only two occupations were licensed, law and medicine. Shortly after the *Dent* v. *West Virginia* decision in 1889, ten occupations were licensed under a total of 110 different state licensure laws. The next two decades saw a doubling of occupations to twenty-one and laws to 195. A steady increase saw thirty occupations licensed in 1920. Greene (1969) estimated, in a review of state codes, almost 2,800 statutory provisions requiring occupational licenses. In 1982 the *Consumer's Resource Handbook* estimated that there were 1,500 state boards licensing more than 550 professions and occupations.

The process by which occupations become licensed (discussed in chapter 1) led initially to the development of separate administrative boards for each occupation. These decentralized boards have often duplicated each other's efforts. Beginning with Illinois in 1917 and Washington, Pennsylvania, California, and New York in the succeeding twenty years, these states grouped licensing boards together under one director. These actions were often resisted by established professions. The combined boards established budgetary controls, gave directors veto power over separate board actions, created independent hearing offices, and pooled investigating staffs. This is discussed further in chapter 6.

The more political power the associations developed, the more they were able to change licensing laws from those that simply restricted the use of an occupational title to laws that reserved the practice of the occupation only to those holding a valid license. In this way professional associations were able to monopolize practice for their members. The professionalizing of medicine had progressed so quickly that by 1925, about fifty years after the passage of the first medical practice act, all state and federal jurisdictions had enacted medical practice restrictions.

The greater exclusiveness of entry requirements has taken several forms. The apprenticeship system of entry to professional occupations has become almost entirely extinct in its original form. It has survived in an altered state under the auspices of educational institutions in the forms of internships and fellowships. The length of training also increased as a result of accreditation pressures emanating from the professional associations. The basis for professional association dominance over service to the public was largely established by the first quarter of the twentieth century. The present state of professional hegemony, in the words of Gerstl and Jacobs (1976), makes "threats to established patterns of dominance appear minimal" (p. 18).

A CASE STUDY: THE WAR AGAINST THE MIDWIVES

The decline in the American midwife's involvement in the birthing process is not just attributable to enlightenment, new medical discoveries, or to changing tastes, though all three are part of the story. More so, it is the story of how a determined minority of medical men over several hundred years was able to organize itself, inform the public of its point of view, and use education, licensing, and monopolistic power to impose their view on the public. At the same time they were able to restrict the activities of women healers and midwives who had provided health and birthing services for millenia. If these developments had served the interests of the public for better treatment then it would not be the good example it is of the use of power and legal structure to enhance the private interests of professionals. This, then, is an occupational case study of the use of licensing in the professionalization of one occupation at the expense of another.

The Old Order

The midwife role is an ancient one for women who from time immemorial had been expected to learn from their mothers how to heal common illnesses, nurse the sick, and birth babies. These skills were indispensable to survival in any community. The management of birth by midwives is noted in the Bible both in Genesis and Exodus. As a role, it fit into a natural order where life was controlled by the exigencies of nature, the amount of rainfall, or the adequacy of a harvest. Birth was a natural process that required a minimal amount of knowledge and often went unattended. Midwifery was a neighborly service performed by social class equals and ethnic compatriots who spoke the same language. Its effectiveness was based on the warmth, caring, and the personal and professional experiences of an observant and very much present midwife. There was an expectation that there would be a personal relationship between the expectant mother and the midwife. Though men had long been associated with the birthing process when emergencies arose, they were generally excluded on the grounds of propriety. This general state of affairs existed until the thirteenth century in Europe when the universities, the churches, and the guilds began to change the premises underlying healing.

Early Skirmishes

The first skirmish in the war against the midwives did not affect the midwife directly. It concerned female healers and focused on the transformation of healing from a female-dominated neighborly healing role to a male-dominated, commodity-oriented medical service.

Donnison (1977) commented that, prior to the thirteenth century in England, medical practice was open to all regardless of education or training. Graduates of Oxford and Cambridge did have the advantage even then of a type of licensure, granted by virtue of their education, to practice under the title of "physician" or "doctor." But with the development in the thirteenth century of the barber-surgeon guilds came the first regulation of surgical practice in towns where the guild system prevailed. In exchange for guaranteeing standards of entry, training, and practice, the guild's members were granted exclusive rights to practice in the town and its surrounding area and the opportunity to prosecute those practicing without the guild's approval.

English physicians campaigned through the parliament and the courts to remove female healers from practice, asking for laws that would impose fines and imprisonment against women who dared to compete with physicians. The Church, the State, and the medical profession combined forces to hold witch trials to root out the women healers. The campaign against witches reached its height in the late fifteenth and early sixteenth centuries and was mostly directed against women. In an orgy of killing in Europe millions died, and Ehrenreich and English (1978) estimated that "85 percent of those executed [were] old women, young women and children" (p. 35). Their crimes included "providing contraceptive measures, performing abortions, offering drugs to ease the pain of labor" (p. 35). The campaign against witches was justified by the threat of the witches' magic to established religious beliefs. There was irony in that male, university-trained physicians based their practice on scientific "logic," Christian theology, bleeding, guesswork and myth; while women healers used herbal treatments which were effective painkillers, digestive aids, and antiinflammatory agents. The male physicians had access to the levers of power and became the ones who were asked to judge whether illnesses were caused by witchcraft or some naturally occurring circumstance. Women healers did not really have a chance—the situation was rigged against them. They were judged to be witches if they presumed to treat people without having "studied" medicine, yet they were not permitted to study in the only curriculum recognized as "scientific"—the male-dominated universities of the time.

The campaign against urban, educated women healers created a monopoly at this time for the male doctors among the upper classes except for the mid-wives who retained a role with the upper classes until late in the eighteenth century. Ehrenreich and English (1973) pointed out that though the witch hunts failed to stop the lower class female healer, they did succeed in labeling her as superstitious and even malevolent. By so discrediting her among the emerging middle class, the witch campaign paved the way for the major male inroads into midwifery that occurred in the eighteenth century.

This was the first step in the transformation of healing from female to male practitioners and made healing a commodity to be sold on the open market. This step was crucial as it lay the groundwork for much that was to follow as Ehrenreich and English (1978) pointed out.

The historical antagonist of the female lay healer was the male medical professional. The notion of medicine as a *profession* was in some ways an advance over the unexamined tradition of female healing. A profession requires systematic training, and at least in principle, some formal mechanisms of accountability. But a profession is also defined by its *exclusiveness*, and has been since the professions of medicine and law first took form in Medieval Europe. While the female lay healer operated within a network of information-sharing and mutual support, the male professional hoarded up his knowledge as a kind of property, to be dispensed to wealthy patrons or sold on the market as a commodity. His goal was not to spread the skills of healing, but to concentrate them within the elite interest group which the professions came to represent. Thus the triumph of the male medical profession . . . involved the destruction of women's networks of mutual help—leaving women in a position of isolation and dependency—and it established a model of expertism as the preroga-tive of a social elite. [p. 34]

An act of the English parliament in 1512 provided a system of licensing skilled and approved practitioners. It did not mention but apparently included midwives. The act was administered by ecclesiastical authorities as part of the campaign to eliminate witchcraft. All applicants with the exception of university graduates were examined by local bishops who, if they were satisfied, would grant the applicants a license to practice in the diocese. Character witnesses and an oath to avoid sorcery made these procedures into a social control device rather than a guarantee of profes-sional skill. More important, they did legitimize the practice of female midwives, though only for a limited period. In 1616 as part of a campaign for secular regulation of midwives, a group of London midwives requested a charter for a society to control the standards of midwife practice. Referred by the king's privy council to the College of Physicians, a judgment was made that it was neither necessary nor convenient to elevate midwives "to the dignity of a self-governing corporation" (Donnison, 1977, p. 14).

Men began making inroads into midwifery in the early seventeenth century as evidenced by the addition of the term *man-midwife* to the

English language at that time. Male midwives appeared to be reserved for difficult cases. Given the widespread concern about decency and propriety, various strategies were used so the male midwife would not compromise the reputation of the patient or the sanctity of marriage. Men were often required to work in half darkness or work "blind" with their hands under sheets.

Two events occurred in the eighteenth century that were to open up midwifery for men in a dramatic way. About 1720 a British surgeon, Peter Chamberlen, introduced the obstetrical forceps. The forceps permitted the physician to deliver live infants where previously either mother or child would have died. The forceps also shortened the period of labor. The forceps enhanced the position of men in the process as women were not permitted by law, custom, and lack of training to use them. Thirty years later the first lying-in hospitals for the poor of London were established allowing male midwives to gain much additional experience with normal deliveries. Thus it was by the end of the eighteenth century in England the concept of male midwifery was accepted by the upper classes. Women midwives attempted to counter this male invasion, citing commercialism and the dangerous misuse of the forceps but they were discredited for being ignorant and clinging to superstition.

The introduction of male midwives to the United States occurred in 1753 despite protestations that the techniques of the male midwife were dangerous. Marieskind (1980) quoted the editor of the *American Practice of Medicine* who wrote, "prior to the sixteenth century not half the number of women died in childbirth as have died in a like period of time since the advent of the man-midwife" (p. 120). U.S. fashion dictated by 1800, however, that upper and middle class women use the male midwives, following their European counterparts.

The first governmental regulation of midwives in the United States occurred in the French colonies of Louisiana, but it took until 1760 for New York State to examine and license midwives. Other American colonies soon followed the lead of New York.

A Century of Discovery in the United States

The second step in the transformation from midwifery to obstetrics occurred during the nineteenth century and, though not restricted to the United States, tended to center there. A series of medical discoveries and procedures changed birthing from a natural process in the view of the middle and upper classes to a malady that could be controlled by using instruments, drugs, and surgery. Litoff (1978) enumerated these developments as shown in table 4.1.

The exclusion of midwives from the use of new instruments, drugs, and operations; their great difficulty in gaining training and information about the birthing process other than through their traditional informal means; and the efforts of the medical profession to upgrade obstetrical practice

TABLES 4.1. Nineteenth-Century U.S. Medical Discoveries in Obstetrics

1808 Ergot introduced to induce uterine contractions.
1809 First successful ovariotomy was performed.
1820s Stethoscope was applied to a woman's abdomen to monitor the fetal heartbeat.
      Instrument to dilate the cervix was introduced.
1840s Introduction of the use of ether for both difficult and normal labors.
      Discovery that puerperal fever was contagious and was carried by way of
        the hands of the attending physician or midwife.
      Introduction of antiseptic techniques.
1850s Curved vaginal speculum was introduced.
      Women's Hospital of New York City opened and was devoted exclusively to
        diseases of women and children.
1860s Clitoridectomy performed in the United States.
1870s Silver nitrate applied to the eyes of newborn infants to prevent ophthalmice
        neonatorum.

Source: Judy B. Litoff, *American Midwives: 1860 to the Present* (Westport, Conn.: Greenwood
    Press, 1978), pp. 18-20.

through specialization all served to raise the status of the physicians
practicing obstetrics and to discredit the work of midwives. Medical schools
were a male preserve until the last half of the nineteenth century, so that the
source of potential knowledge was effectively cut off from the mass of
female midwives. Even after the inclusion of women in medical education as
late as 1973 Ehrenreich and English (1973) reported that only 7 percent of
America's doctors were women and only 13 percent of medical students
were women (Marieskind, 1980). The efforts of some physicians to provide
education and training for midwives were opposed by the medical establishment fearful of competition and of legitimizing "second-class obstetrical
care." (Marieskind, 1980, p. 121).

These developments had an impact primarily on the middle and upper
classes. During the middle half of the nineteenth century, a popular health
movement attracted many adherents among working class and rural people.
The United States saw the softening or actual repeal of restrictive medical-
licensing laws. A part of the larger egalitarian social movement, it was to
be the last time midwives would have strong support for their perspective.
Samuel Thomson and the Thomsonians took the lead in opposing "heroic"
obstetrical practices.

Thomson himself strongly disapproved of male, regular obsetrical practice. The
doctors were less experienced than midwives, he argued (at this time most regular
physicians received their degrees without having witnessed a delivery), and too

prone to rush things with the forceps, a practice which often resulted in crushed or deformed babies. [Ehrenreich and English, 1978, p. 53]

The popular health movement eventually broke up into warring cults, dissipating its egalitarian social energy and with it the remaining prestige and socially acceptable justifications for midwifery. These developments left the midwives vulnerable to assault by the obstetricians who in the last quarter of the nineteenth century prepared for the final campaign against them.

The Final Campaign

At the dawn of the twentieth century, midwives were aiding in the births of only 50 percent of America's babies, primarily from poor, working class, and immigrant families. The next thirty years was a period during which midwifery would be outlawed or ignored and turned into an officially despised and discredited occupation peopled, it was said, by the dirty, the ignorant, and the incompetent. The rhetoric of scientific medicine and the reality of medical practice were actually at odds. Ehrenreich and English (1978) reported (1) that physicians were not prepared to replace the midwives they were proposing to eliminate, there not being "enough obstetricians in the United States to serve the masses of poor and working class women, even if the obstetricians were inclined to do so" (p. 97); (2) that obstetricians introduced a new danger into the birthing process, inclined as they were to intervene with knife or forceps if the going was too slow for their schedule; and (3) that, according to a 1911 study "most American doctors at the time were *less* competent than the midwives they were replacing . . . less experienced . . . less observant, and less likely to even be *present* at a critical moment" (p. 97). Litoff (1978) quoting from the same 1911 study revealed that, "general practitioners lose as many and possibly more women from puerperal infection than do midwives" (p. 65).

Over time, however, the physicians' rhetoric influenced policy decisions which, in turn, influenced the reality of practice. The means by which this was accomplished was discussed earlier in this chapter as so-called scientific medicine reformed the practice of medicine in America, eliminating "unscientific" medical education and the cults they supported. The opening shot was to differentiate obstetrics from midwifery, these two terms having been used interchangeably prior to the twentieth century. Thus obstetrics firmed up its link with traditional medicine. Continued interpretation of childbirth as a pathological problem was essential to the campaign against midwives. It rationalized requiring pregnant women to be confined and indisposed throughout their nine-month term (to avoid all stimulation so as not to stunt or deform their babies) and to accept a protracted period of convalescence.

It was essential to the campaign to exorcise the midwives that they be seen as ignorant and dirty. Since there had been a continuing refusal in this country to train midwives, the discoveries of the eighteenth and nineteenth centuries were not made available to most midwives so there was a basis for the charges made against them. Where competent training was made available, it made a difference. This was the European solution to the problem. According to Litoff (1978), the English Midwives Act of 1902, which involved the training of midwives, reduced English infant mortality from 151 deaths per 1,000 live births in 1901 to 106 deaths per 1,000 live births in 1910. In another example, New York City established a Bureau of Child Hygiene in 1908 to supervise the activities of midwives and to create a school for midwives. The infant mortality rate in 1907 was 144 deaths per 1,000 live births and was reduced in 1921 to 71.1 deaths per 1,000 live births. Litoff's (1978) report concludes, "Certainly, the training and supervision of New York's midwives, who attended between 26 and 40 percent of the births in the city from 1910 to 1920, was a significant factor in bringing about this decline" (p. 93). But on the whole the American solution was to outlaw and ignore them. While in Europe the result was better care for pregnant women, in America the result was the triumph of the physician over the midwife and the creation of a medical monopoly.

Litoff (1978) indicated that the campaign against midwives reached its height between 1910 and 1920. By 1910 midwives were attending 40.55 percent of all births but by 1920 the figure shrank to 26.6 percent. In the state of New Jersey between 1911 and 1920 the number of practicing midwives was reduced by 56 percent. Even more dramatic, midwives in Birmingham, Alabama, attended 968 births in 1917 but only 10 in 1924. This trend did not extend to rural areas. Rural midwives were the only service available to pregnant women because of the severe shortage of physicians, poor transportation, and lack of facilities.

The campaign against the midwives centered on the development of obstetrics as a viable medical specialty. The assumption motivating activity suppressing midwives was that their very existence was an obstacle to the development of the specialty (midwives were a significant economic competitor and their practice kept fees lower than other areas of medical practice) and they stood as a symbol of the inadequacies of obstetrical practice. The success of the campaign was assured by continuing technological innovations (for example, painless child birth, the prophylactic forceps operation, and marked increased use of the caesarean operation) which convinced more Americans to view childbirth as a pathology. This in turn supported the building of hospitals and the provision in them for childbirth, which in turn supported the increased use of more heroic interventions, the acceptance by even more persons of the pathology view, and the choice of the physician over the midwife. All of this occurred during a time of a strong Americanization and "melting pot" spirit abroad in the land. Midwives had their greatest support among the immigrants in the cities and among the black poor in the South. Midwifery was identified with foreigners and the racially downtrodden, another support for the increasing turn to physicians for those with an option. The period started out with 50 percent of the births in America attended in 1900 by midwives ended with only 15 percent so attended by 1930. Litoff (1978) described the social factors responsible: (1) the decline in immigration, (2) the decline in the birth rate, (3) the availability of easy transportation (auto) to hospitals, (4) the perception of birth as a special event and a complex medical disorder, and (5) the perception by many women of the hospital as a rest from household chores.

The Aftermath

Where the activities of physicians and midwives have been monitored, physicians compared unfavorably. A 1933 study by the New York Academy of Medicine, reported by Litoff (1978), of 2,041 maternal deaths between 1930 and 1933 judged two-thirds to have been preventable. Physicians were held responsible for 61 percent, midwives 2 percent, and patient judgment for 27 percent. Though it is true that physicians get the more difficult cases, that does not entirely explain the difference in maternal death rate: surgeons are involved in 9.9 deaths per 1,000 live births; obstetricians in 5.4; and midwives in 1.4. Another study in 1932, reported by Litoff (1978) showed that "at the international level there was a definite relationship between low maternal mortality and high percentage of births attended by midwives" (p. 109). Too great a recourse by physicians to forceps, anesthesia, and the caesarean operation was blamed.

The poor showing of the United States when compared internationally despite a cost of health care that outstrips all other countries continues long after obstetrics has been accepted as a specialty and most births occur in hospitals. Litoff (1978) places the United States as sixth (18.5 deaths per 1,000 live births) when compared in 1972 to Sweden (10.7), the Netherlands (11.7), Norway (11.8), Denmark (12.2), and England (17.2). She noted that the countries that were superior to the United States had (1) midwives (both lay and nurse) as a part of a health care team, (2) more conservative birthing practices, and (3) government-sponsored insurance programs. Another result is that there was almost an absence of maternal death in Denmark, Norway, and Sweden, while the U.S. rate was 1.5 deaths per 1,000 live births. Litoff concluded: "It is unfortunate that Americans have been so reluctant to endorse the concept of the midwife. It is quite likely that the present infant and maternal mortality rate of the United States would compare more favorably with other modern industrial nations if properly educated midwives and nurse-midwives were utilized to their fullest extent" (p. 147).

The trend toward the use of the hospital has continued in the United States to the point that it completely dominates the market. Marieskind (1980) reported that the number of Caucasian babies born in hospitals went from 60 percent in 1940 to 99 percent in 1977, while "all others" went from 27 percent in 1940 to 98 percent in 1977. Only 64,000 babies were born outside of a hospital in the United States each year in recent years. Since physicians control the hospital, they control the birthing process. The war is over. The lay midwife has just about disappeared from the scene. Twenty-five states still have midwife licensure laws on the books but most do not implement them. There is a flicker of interest from those following alternative life styles and those utilizing self-help, holistic, and alternative health modalities. The natural childbirth movement and the nurse-midwife may yet restore the positive values associated with the older order but their influence is still minor. Nurse-midwives are licensed in forty-eight states, but they are not allowed to receive third-party payments from insurance companies nor are they allowed hospital privileges for problem births. Physicians who cooperate with nurse-midwives as a backup for emergencies are ostracized by other physicians in some communities. Cooperation between physicians and midwives is blocked presently because state medical societies refuse to support malpractice insurance programs for physicians assisting in home deliveries. The war is over. The midwives are routed. Physicians are in firm control of the birthing process.

5

THE PROFESSIONS
AND LICENSING

The organization of occupations into the modern professions has been an important consequence of the age of enlightenment in the eighteenth century and the industrial revolution of the nineteenth century. These developments caused a break with past forms of occupational organization as new ways of organizing knowledge and relationships were required (Houle, 1980). Occupations are ways of organizing knowledge, thus professions are a modern adaptation of this function.

Stewart and Cantor (1974) noted two reasons sociologists have been so interested in the professions. With ever more specialization of knowledge, there have been an increasing number of attempts of many occupations to professionalize. Some sociologists wonder if the whole labor force is to become professionalized. The major professions also exert a great deal of influence in their responsibility for critical aspects of communal life and receive the perquisites of rewards, prestige, and political power. Underlying this interest is the influence of numbers. The proportion that professionals and related occupations were of the total American labor force more than trebled between 1900 and 1970 (from 4.3 percent to 14.2 percent according to Collins's [1979] interpretation of census data). Houle (1980) also examined census data for the period between 1910 and 1976. Finding a similar increase of professionals in the proportion of the work force, he showed a 660-percent increase in the number of persons employed as professionals during a time when the work force increased only 135 percent.

With increasing numbers, power, and prestige comes increasing visibility. Houle (1980) noted that since 1965 the inadequacies of the professions have stimulated increasing alarm and disillusionment. Explaining this as the unintended consequences of rapid growth and the failure of systems designed for smaller associations, he noted three criticisms. One criticism focused on the perceived failure of professionals to service the entire population, especially the poor and the alienated. A second centered on the perceived pursuit of self-interest rather than community interest by many professionals. A third was the accusation that professional practices "demonstrate incompetence, inattention, dogmatism, lack of feeling, or malevolence" (p. 27). Begun (1980) supported this in the introduction to his study of professional quality: "In the minds of many citizens today . . . professionalism is a word that connotes elitism, exclusion, and exploitation. Professions are seen as grasping, careless elite groups responsible to no one, rather than altruistic groups of experts whose ethics ensure the quality of their services at a fair price" (p. 1). Houle (1980) is careful to point out that such charges may have as much to do with the increases in the power and influence of professions as with the general state of practice in professions, but they do indicate the kinds of problems needing attention in any future restoration of public confidence in the professions.

Lenrow's (1978) analysis indicated that the problem of the professions cannot be separated from other problems in our highly mobile and increasingly anonymous society. He contrasts two types of helping relationships—*aid to strangers in distress* and *long-term social exchange.* The former is characterized by service to persons outside the helper's usual social network in a temporary relationship where the helper has great power which is used to help the outsider without prospects of reciprocity. On the other hand, long-term social exchange occurs where the service is to known persons who are part of the helper's network of reciprocal obligations. The service is part of a complex series of social interactions characterized by cooperation, sharing, mutual benefits, and a long-term common fate. Citing studies showing increasing tendencies for American society to be characterized as a "nation of strangers" living in temporary relationships and in fragmented social networks and vanishing neighborhoods, he concluded, "the conditions for help as long-term social exchange are becoming more and more rare" (p. 272). Contrasting the rural and urban stereotypes of the professional role he, in effect, suggested an explanation for the criticism of professional helpers as self-serving, arbitrary, dogmatic, manipulative, and aloof as a response to the loss or lack of integration of the professional's life with the life of clients outside the helping role. The helper involved in long-term social exchange is "subject to social control by the community, including clients, through everyday interactions [as opposed to] regulations by bureaucratic organizations that license, ensure, and pay him and lobby on behalf of his profession" (p. 273).

THE PURPOSES OF PROFESSIONS

The characteristics attributed to professions as ideal types and in practice vary quite a bit. Barber (1965) explained that indistinctness is maintained because the term *professional* carries "an important assignment of differential occupational prestige" (p. 17). There are a variety of purposes and interests involved in particular definitions. The term is used both in an evaluative as well as in a descriptive manner. Occupational groups use the terms "to flatter themselves or try to persuade others of their importance . . . [thus] it is hopeless to expect the word to refer to more than a social symbol differentially applied" (Freidson, 1970, p. 4). For Freidson (1970) it is "folly to be dogmatic about any definition of 'professions' or to assume that its definition is so well known that it warrants no discussion" (p. 4). Barber (1965) believed: "There is no absolute difference between professional and other kinds of occupational behavior, but only relative differences with respect to certain attributes common to all occupational behavior" (p. 17).

The next section will identify these attributes, though even here there is not complete agreement. This lack of agreement explains the difficulty encountered by the Quebec government's *L'Office des Professions* in implementing its new code. The code distinguished particular professions entitled to charters granting them "exclusive right of practice" from those granted charters allowing "reserve of title." The problem was posed by the sixty-eight occupations not named in the code that filed requests for charters or made inquiry about charters. Bureaucratic decision making, rather than the interest-group politics of the United States, was necessitated. They found that "the exact boundary that separates the professions from other occupations is difficult to draw with precision. . . . [T]he specifications in the law for a profession are difficult to apply and are not useful for a decision in a specific case. Even if a professional cannot be sharply defined, almost everybody in Quebec wants to be one" (Bosk, 1977, p. 68).

It follows from this introduction that the definition of professions would somehow beg the question of clarifying their nature. Larson (1977) described professions as "occupations with special power and prestige . . . [which] tend to become 'real' communities, whose members share a relatively permanent affiliation, an identity, personal commitment, specific interests, and general loyalties" (p. 4).

To gain an appreciation for the purpose of professions one must consider their historical function. Earlier, the primary function of professions—that of organizing knowledge—was identified. Larson (1977) identified two secondary functions, one economic and one social. The economic purpose emerged as a consequence of the opportunities gained for earning a living as a result of the industrial revolution and the consolidation of capitalism. The new importance of the market at that time "created new areas of practice and new occupational roles. The application of science to industry and to practically every other area of life gradually and constantly changed the cognitive bases of the social division of labor" (p. 17). Professional work became a new way of earning a livelihood as a response to changing economic and social conditions in the eighteenth and nineteenth centuries. These developments were related to and occurred at a time of decline in the aristocratic tradition, so the professions tended to be populated by the social elite as a way of guaranteeing their status and credibility.

Collins (1979) explained the modern professional movement, which began in the late nineteenth century in the United States, as a response to

the breaking down of the closed corporate controls of the traditional professions and a general democratization of occupational access. The shift back to professionalism began in the atmosphere of a nativist counterattack in the late nineteenth century against the influx of culturally alien immigration and political reform in defense of the local powers of the Anglo-Protestant middle class. [p. 13]

Professions then became institutions to conserve the powers of an elite class at a time when the prior sources of power were diminishing. In this regard, Larson (1977) suggested an underlying social control purpose: "Viewed in the larger perspective of the occupational and class structures, it would appear that the model of profession passes from a predominantly economic function—organizing the linkage between education and marketplace—to a predominantly ideological one—justifying inequality of status and closure of access in the occupational order" (p. xviii). The maintenance of privilege is thus suggested as an underlying secondary function of professions. This perspective was supported by Ehrenreich and Ehrenreich (n.d.) who postulated a professional-managerial class of "mental workers who did not own the means of production" (p. 67) and who were dedicated to the reproduction of the class through lengthy training. This social function led Larson (1977) to suggest that "Professions are not exclusively occupational categories: whatever else they are professions are situated in the middle and upper middle levels of the stratification system. Both objectively and subjectively, professions are outside and above the working class, as occupations and as social strata" (p. xvi).

ATTRIBUTES OF PROFESSIONS

One way to contain the booming, buzzing confusion of professional phenomena is to set out the central characteristics in an abstract and ideal form. Lenrow (1978) defined the "enduring ideals" associated with the professional role.

These are the values of impartiality, rationality, empirical knowledge, and ethics committed to the dignity of the individual and to the public welfare. . . . *Impartial* does not mean morally neutral but instead means dispassionate and fair, rather than self-serving. *Rational* means reflective and attentive to the logic and the persuasiveness of alternative arguments, rather than impulsive or arbitrary. *Empirical knowledge* here means beliefs based on experience and open to correction on the basis of new experiences, rather than held with a closed mind. *Respect for the dignity of the individual* means abstaining from covert or coercive manipulation of people as means to one's own ends. And *commitment to public welfare* means taking into account in one's actions what would promote just or healthy interrelationships of all groups, rather than working blindly for a special interest group conceived of in isolation from the rest of the community. [pp. 268-69]

Since life does not conveniently fit abstract categories, it is useful to judge the extent to which an occupation is professionalized on the basis of the degree to which the formal attributes of professions apply. Goode (1960) pointed out that the attributes of a profession were highly interdependent with one another. As factors in social relationships they identified a system of rights and obligations among clients, professionals, and external agencies. An occupation was professionalized by a process of gradual development, clarification, internalization, and crystallization of role relationships within the profession and between the profession and the remainder of the society. The following attributes represent, at the least, the role expectations in the ideal and, at the best, the role performances seen more rarely in practice, which are involved in the behavior and institutions we label as professional. Five attributes emerge from a sifting of the treatises on professions: calling, knowledge, association, autonomy, and altruism.

A Sense of Calling

With obvious throwback to earlier times when professionals were priests or military officers, a calling refers to an understanding of the motive to work at a profession—in this case an inner sense that an occupation is especially appropriate for the individual almost to the extent that he or she *must* do it or has been asked to do it by some higher authority. Where a sense of calling exists, members are strongly identified with their profession; they work at it full time (or more), derive from it their principal source of income, and make a deep and usually lifetime commitment to it. Such a profession experiences a low turnover ratio. A sense of calling may be contrasted with monetary rewards when comparing motivation for an occupation or profession.

A Body of Knowledge

Professions are based on the availability of a particular and useful body of knowledge developed as the result of a highly intellectual process. Knowledge may have profound consequences for practical affairs; consequently, professionals are given a great deal of authority and responsibility for its appropriate use. This knowledge is not made available to the public, remaining esoteric so the skills of utilizing it may be monopolized and the public kept dependent on a limited number of professionals. Professions attempt to achieve a "monopoly of credibility" (Larson, 1977, p. 17) so as to maintain their hold on the knowledge and the upper hand in their relationship with the public and with competing professionals.

The need of professions to maintain their knowledge monopoly makes professional ideologies, according to Freidson (1973), "intrinsically imperialistic, claiming more for the profession's knowledge and skill, and a broader jurisdiction, than can in fact be justified by demonstrable effectiveness" (p. 31). Professional claims rest on a particular (to each profession) and yet all-inclusive view of their world, which is highly resistant to change. Professionals tend to confer on their view a "taken-for-granted," true believer, or absolutistic quality. As a result professions may compete with one another for jurisdiction over particular phenomena, procedures, and so on, arguing in favor of their particular definition of the problem or ways of solving it. Thus, professionals argue, only those who have been properly inducted into the world view and the knowledge base are capable of judging another professional's practice. Extensive training under the control of the profession—involving the knowledge core, the esoteric services and skills, and a socialization process that develops appropriate attitudes in aspiring professionals—is required and a connection is usually made to the modern seats of learning, the universities. According to Lieberman (1970), one of the consequences of this special status is the permission "to do dangerous things, to talk about things in a shocking way, to do what others would not dare [to] hear the inner torments of disturbed men and women [or] build bridges which the public will cross" (p. 56).

Hughes (1965) pointed out that professionals have permission to deviate from lay conduct in regard to these matters, "they profess to know better than others [and are] expected to think objectively and inquiringly about matters which may be for laymen, subject to orthodoxy and sentiment which limit intellectual exploration" (p. 2). Detachment is a characteristic professional behavior that involves finding "an intellectual base for the problems one handles, which, in turn, takes those problems out of their particular setting and makes them part of some universal order" (p. 6). In occupations that have not emerged into full professional status, the knowledge base may be diffuse in the sense that it is shared with other occupations or the public; it is unevenly distributed among members of the occupations so that many members can only do what they are told to do; or it is clearly inadequate to the task of dealing with the problems of practicing the occupation.

A Formal Organization

The maintenance of a monopoly of knowledge requires a community in which cooperation among members and restraints on their behavior may promote the common interest of the group and protect them from the incursions of others. The association is essentially voluntary and operated by the members themselves. It is collegial in character, a horizontal collection of equals in contrast to the vertical and hierarchical bureaucratic organization. The organization confers admission, reputation, and the very warrant to practice the profession either directly—most highly professionalized occupations control practice through state licensing—or indirectly by providing a symbol for the public to understand that the profession has a unique body of knowledge and skill. The organization provides a clear reference group as the source of ideas, models, and judgments. The values of noncompetitiveness preserve the unity of the organization, while altruism justifies the special perquisites the profession receives. Altruism also wards off external attempts to regulate the members, which, if allowed, could destroy the organization by robbing it of its reward and permission-granting powers. Less professionalized occupations may lack a clear identity for their members or the power to gain their actual membership in the professional community and the authority to regulate their members' behavior. As a result they present a more diffuse picture to the public.

A High Degree of Autonomy

The result of a self-regulating profession is a high degree of discretion reserved for the members over the decisions relevant to practice. This is made appropriate in the public's mind by the esoteric base of knowledge that outsiders are not believed to be able to competently judge.

Friedson (1973) indicated that professionals "tend to believe that their work is of such a complex character, requiring so much judgment, that formal standards or rules are too arbitrary to be applicable. Typically, they insist on individual discretion, denying the possibility and propriety of formal rules" (p. 34). Professionals assume the right to define error or failure and resent public discussion of professional mistakes as a threat to their autonomy. Professionals rarely criticize one another for fear they will be criticized in return and because the knowledge is made so esoteric that precise definitions of mistakes do not appear to exist. Distance between professionals and the public is maintained by condescending attitudes, patronizing behavior, and resistance, manipulation, tokenism, or co-optation in response to any possibility of sharing decision-making authority. The professional is rendered immune from client control by maintaining the power to define the client's needs, for as Lieberman (1970) explained "The client who defines any needs would be in a position to control the professional's actions and ultimately thus to usurp his function" (p. 59). It follows that the professional takes responsibility for defining what public policy should be toward the profession. A license is a mandate that signifies the agreement of the society and validates the claims to status and autonomy. The consequence, according to Hughes (1965), is that: "The true professional . . . is never hired. He is retained, engaged, consulted, etc., by someone who has need of his services. He, the professional, has or should have almost complete control over what he does for the client" (p. 9). The lesser degree of discretion or control over practice differentiates the occupations from the professions with the public, clients, or employers thus having greater opportunity for decision making about the nature and quality of practice by occupation members.

An Altruistic Attitude

An altruistic attitude is exemplified by the goal of service to the community as opposed to individual self-interest. Professionals espouse a system of self-regulation that uses standards embodied in a code of ethics to encourage exemplary behavior by the members of the profession. Collins (1979) pointed to the source of the altruistic attitude: "The elite professions in America grew out of older gentry elites; their communal organization from upper-class clients and their legitimating ideology from the traditions of upper-class altruism and religious leadership" (p. 135). *Noblesse oblige* refers to the obligation that those of high social rank have to be honorable, generous, and responsible. The obligation of a service orientation—accenting how beneficial and indispensable the service is to the community—has its roots in upper-class generosity rhetoric and justifies the consumer protection argument central to the delegation of police power. The image portrayed is of selfless dedication to the community good and of ethical restraints that encourage service-oriented attitudes—to do no harm, to act in the client's interest, and to protect the client's confidence. Lieberman (1970) pointed out that professionals cultivate an attitude of neutrality, which requires them to act altruistically whether they feel that way or not. The professional "professes a desire to serve all and to serve to the maximum of his ability, regardless of the size of his compensation or other material reward. The professional asserts that the skills he has to offer are actually or potentially beneficial to all (p. 57). According to Hughes (1965),

Since the professional does profess, he asks to be trusted. . . . A central feature, then, of all professions is the motto—not used in this form, so far as I know—*credat emptor.* This is the professional relation distinguished from that of those markets in which the rule is *caveat emptor.* . . . [T]he client is to trust the professional; he must tell him all secrets which bear upon the affairs in hand. He must trust his judgment and skill. [pp. 2-3]

There is great disparity between the image and the reality. But the images are powerful and support the mystique of selfless, dedicated service, despite the little effort expended to restrain professionals from financial exploitation, the failure of self-control, and the use of self-regulation to control competition and insure monopoly. Professionals appear to behave similarly to nonprofessionals with regard to self-interest and self-control but may be distinguished by their stated ideals which are discussed as if they were fully realized. In understanding the nature of this phenomenon it is helpful to view the professions in light of their guildlike qualities.

PROFESSION AS GUILD

Benham (1980) indicated that guilds were a form of association and regulated workers from the time they were first noted in London in the tenth century until the eighteenth century. Seeing some striking similarities between the guild and the modern licensed occupation, Benham said: "the impulse to regulate occupations through licensure or its equivalent has been widespread, and the resulting associations have shown strong survival traits. In this regard, the nineteenth century, which saw a decline in guild influence, appears to have been an anomaly. During the present century, the United States appears to be reverting to the norm" (p. 13). Carman (1958) noted that the association between the historic professions and the Church-controlled medieval university made professionals "a class apart" (p. 269). Emerging from the domination of the church, medical professionals formed associations in England in the sixteenth century, "which evolved into guilds" (p. 269). Pharmacists, architects, dentists, engineers, and accountants followed a similar path.

Gerstl and Jacobs (1976) described a craft guild as follows: "They restricted competition, set prices, defined the quality of raw materials and craftsmanship, controlled entrance and training, and generally developed ordinances touching on the guildsman's relations with fellow members, non-members, members of other guilds, future members, dependent workers, and consumers" (p. 2).

Brown and Cassady (1947) noted the modern elaboration of the earlier craft guild.

Perhaps the outstanding feature of the development of modern guilds is the manner in which their growth has been secured by legislative action. Lacking this endorsement, associations of members of a trade might run afoul of a state antitrust legislation, if they attempted to agree upon such matters as minimum prices, working hours and the right to practice the occupation. But these same associations have prevailed upon legislatures of many states to "protect the public welfare" by passing laws which accomplish the same result. [pp. 312-13]

Though Brown and Cassady were referring to barbers and other service tradespeople, the analogy is applicable to professional associations. The ways in which professionals are socialized and the restrictions on entry to professional occupations work to forge similar, though implicit, agreements on prices, working conditions, and incomes.

Professionals may wish to deny any similarity between their associations and guilds because of the crass commercialism or the association with unionism suggested by the guild label. Gilb (1966) suggested this similarity was an oversimplification. Though resembling the medieval institution, she notes that professions are held together more by bureaucratic rules, rational laws, and money symbols than by custom and personal loyalty. There is a vast difference too in the extent to which member behavior is regulated. The analogy, nonetheless, is helpful in understanding the centrality of licensing to professional practice and to account for the high survival value of licensed occupations and their deep historical roots. The charter of autonomy is given to the professional via the licensing arrangement on the basis of public acceptance of the ideas of professional expertise and altruism (Haug and Sussman, 1969). The charter is essential. Without it, professionals would not be able to control the potentially shareable knowledge that is the basis of their expertise, nor would they bother to guide practitioners to make the costly pretense of the altruistic ideal (Haug and Sussman, 1969; Reiff, 1974). To maintain the charter, the professional must mystify the public by making the service appear to be expert and altruistic.

Modern professionals conceal their commercial interests, but these are nonetheless apparent in professional procedures. Reiff (1974) described the professional entrepreneur dealing with knowledge as a commodity, "supplying and withholding for a price service as a form of labor" (p. 455). Carlson's (1975) opinion was that "Health is no longer a condition. It is a commodity, a unique nonfungible good . . . a concomitant of the professionalization of providers who are no longer healers but sellers of goods chopped into units of health" (p. 194). The process of making professional knowledge a commodity requires some sleight of hand. Larson (1977) pointed out that professional work was only a fictitious commodity since professionals did not produce goods; their product was tied to the producer. Therefore, "the producers themselves have to be produced" (p. 14), by which Larson meant professionals must be socialized to provide clearly distinct services. These services were then standardized to establish their superiority "to clearly differentiate their identity and connect them, in the minds of consumers, with stable criteria of evaluation" (p. 14). According to Krause (1977), for physicians, "the key variable is power gained through possession of the medical skill. The power is legitimized—made official—through licensing laws which prohibit others from practicing medicine" (p. 35). But it is not knowledge itself that gives the power, As Freidson (1973) has said, "only *exclusive* knowledge gives power to its possessors" (p. 28). Larson (1977) indicated that "Professional entrepreneurs . . . were, therefore, bound to solicit state protection and state-enforced penalties against unlicensed competitors" (p. 14) to make credible their claim to "sole control of superior expertise" (p. 13).

Controlling the knowledge, making it a commodity, creates a scarcity economy over which the professionals have monopolistic control. Though there is talk about a free market, "health care providers themselves are not responsive to market pressures exerted by consumers, because demand levels are not determined by consumers but by physicians" (Carlson, 1970, p. 857). The accepted sequence of market behavior from consumer to market to producer is reversed so that "consumer demand is increasingly less important in stimulating production than producers are in stimulating consumer demand" (Lieberman, 1970, p. 59). Evidence for this phenomenon is provided by Stevens (1982) who indicated that "areas with a surplus of physicians show an eight-fold increase in the use of medical services and a four-fold increase in surgical services compared to areas matched demographically but without a physician surplus" (p. 246).

By having control over the spigot, professionals can arrange things so that they are benefited rather than their clients. For example, Carlson (1970) pointed to the choice of a fee-for-service system as opposed to a prepayment system. In a fee-for-service system, services, "the need for which is determined by the providers of those services, are continuously bought by users" (p. 858). According to Carlson, this induced inelasticity in demand by restricting user choice and led to increases in costs. The alternative, prepayment, gave providers and consumers a common goal—maintenance of health. Krause (1977) pointed out that in a fee-for-service system it is to the physician's economic advantage to overdefine who is ill, while in a prepayment system it is advantageous to underdefine this group. There is a sleight of hand operating here that Lieberman (1970) described.

the professional scorns the practice of capitalism in order to practice it faithfully. . . . [W]hile the professional claims to serve the public interest and be concerned not one whit about his own interest . . . and while the professional is respectable, responsible, and redoubtable, he is actually behaving in a remarkable capitalistic manner. The professional is the last of the entrepreneurs; like the robber barons before him, he is merely trying to work through the market to monopoly. [p. 137]

The charter of autonomy, given by legislative act, permits regulated occupations to refuse to accept grievance procedures not under their own control. It includes the authority to define the terms of practice and "a legal, moral, and intellectual mandate to determine for the individual and society at large what is healthy, moral, ethical, deviant, normal, or abnormal" (Reiff, 1974, p. 452). With each professional reserving the right to define a mistake or a failure, it follows that professionals rarely criticize each other and that there is little effort put into defining precise standards so that others can make such a judgment. Thus, a system of logic and perception may be erected that organizes ethics and rationalization to protect professionals from the effects of their decisions. Professionals are in a position where they do not suffer the consequences of their own decisions. Recently, even that standard remedy, the malpractice suit, was muted by most state legislatures, which limited the size of awards, lawyers' fees, and times for filing complaints. Those dependent on professionals suffer from their mistakes, ignorance, self-deception, and bias, since professionals have the right (indeed, the mandate) to define when a mistake has been made. In this way a situation is created in which feedback from experience is so limited that self-corrective action is unlikely.

These trappings of power led Gerstl and Jacobs (1976) to observe the "shift of emphasis on the part of professionals from control over the quality of the product or service to control of price" (p. 9). Such power is widely emulated, so much so that many want their occupations to become professions. Gerstl and Jacobs observed that the mystique of the professional is considered so socially useful for so many purposes that there is no consideration that it could be a liability.

DEPENDENCY AND PROFESSIONALS

One explanation for the public's dependency and mystification is that it has been deliberately nurtured by professionals. Another is that it is a natural outgrowth of the importance of knowledge in modern society that professionals have used for their own self-interest. Bledstein (1976), citing the first reason, viewed professionals as using their special knowledge about potential disasters to reduce the client to a state of desperation, engendering the client's willingness to "pay generously, cooperate fully and express undying loyalty to the knowledgeable patron who might save him from a threatening universe" (p. 100). The culture of professionalism, according to Bledstein, "bred public attitudes of submission and passivity" (p. 104) by cultivating an atmosphere of constant crisis, "in which practitioners both created work for themselves and reinforced their authority by intimidating clients" (p. 100). Tennov (1975) cited an especially pertinent example.

The warning that "psychotic episodes" can be precipitated by people who "do not know what they are doing" has been issued again and again over the past seventy years to protect the therapist's monopolization of treatment. The tremendous authority vested in the highly trained and licensed professional makes it more likely that if harm is to be done, it will be he who does it. [p. 140]

Bledstein (1976) described the impact of this use of professional knowledge on public attitudes: "Common sense, ordinary understanding, and personal negotiations no longer were the effective means of human communication in society, as the old-fashioned egalitarian had once thought they should be. Now clients found themselves compelled to believe on simple faith that a higher rationality called scientific knowledge decided one's fate" (p. 94).

Krause (1977) saw the same result, but as a consequence of increasing technological complexity so that "the functional power of expertise lies in the fact that it is a necessity" (p. 237). Knowledge is hoarded; it is made esoteric rather than popularized; and, rather than being used for the good of all, it is appropriated by special interest groups and used for their own benefit. To further complicate matters, the professional was formerly responsible as an agent in relationship to the client. The information explosion, technological advances, and bureaucratization of professional services have corrupted this relationship to the extent that the professional's loyalties are now often determined by the professional's reference group or bureaucratic sponsor or both (Mechanic, 1976). Clients in bureaucratic service organizations are less confident in themselves because of the new territory in which they find themselves and because they are separated—by organizational procedures, informational control, and confusion about where decisions are made—from participating in decision making about the service affecting them (Krause, 1977).

LICENSING AS THE KEY TO PROFESSIONAL POWER

It has been observed that licensing has rarely been sought by the public; rather, it has been sought by the professionals who wished to be licensed (Cohen, 1975; Friedman, 1962). In effect, the legal mechanisms of the State legitimize the occupation. Freidson (1970) observed:

The foundation on which the analysis of a profession must be based is its relationship to the ultimate source of power and authority in modern society—the state. In the case of medicine, much, though by no means all, of the profession's strength is based on legally supported monopoly over practice. This monopoly operates through a system of licensing that bears on the privilege to hospitalize patients and the right to prescribe drugs and order laboratory procedures that are otherwise virtually inaccessible. [p. 83]

Hardcastle (1977) called the need for legal protection an "expedient of an occupation on the make" (p. 14). The occupation becomes "made," ironically, as a profession through the use of public institutions and in opposition to the public interest. Friedman (1962) called the results of licensing "unendurable," even in medicine where the case for licensing is the strongest.

Carlson (1970) described licensing as going from a presumed remedy to a problem: "Licensure would likely fall of its own weight except for a reverence for professionalism" (p. 860). Licensure statutes are defended vigorously by the professions because their loss would mean the loss of a captured board that acts in their interest and the loss of the power as a result of making the violation of the professional monopoly punishable as a crime. So licensure is vitally important to the professionals.

On the other hand, the public is gullible (Moore, 1961), loosely organized, and lacking expertise when compared to the highly motivated trade and professional groups (Shimberg, 1976). In this regard, Krause (1977) observed that the public does not judge expertise. Technically incompetent general practitioners have as many patients as competent ones. The conclusion is thus made by many that the public cannot protect itself and that licensing is, therefore, a necessity.

The complex structure surrounding licensing permits professionals to hide their dependence on the licensing statute from the public's view. According to Freidson (1970), the barrier to freedom to choose practitioners, which is created by licensing, is the foundation of the entire system of service. There are several professions (for example, scientists, university professors, librarians) that are not licensed, usually because they practice in institutions. Goode (1960) suggested that pressure for licensing was greatest for occupations that dealt with clients as individuals and where competence could not easily be demonstrated.

More than 100 years ago it was recognized that the licensing laws had provided the professions with their power, so it was these laws that became the target for attack (Tabachnik, 1976). This may not happen in this century, but it is useful and important to note that the problem of licensing is brought about through the complicity of state governments.

Licensing statutes set up supervisory arrangements by which physician's assistants and nurses, for example, are unable to practice outside of physician control or dental hygienists outside of dentist control. Dolan (1980) pointed out that the physician or dentist controls potential competitors as well as the nature of the competition for their self-interest. "The economics of this situation are appalling. In order for a patient to purchase an auxiliary's services, he or she must first purchase a physician's services. This is a form of mandatory fee splitting. . . ." (pp. 232-33). Since auxiliary personnel can also safely do preventative work (for example, nurse-practitioners—well-baby clinics; optometrists—glaucoma tests; podiatrists —feet maintenance; dental hygienists—cleaning teeth) their turf wars with physicians and dentists have slowed the diffusion of less costly, less intrusive, and potentially more widely effective regimens.

In the 1970s there was a rather strong push to reform licensing laws, for example, national credentialing and institutional licensure (Cohen, 1976; Roemer, 1973). Though it was appealing to believe that there was hope for the system, the facts were that professionals would remain in control in the reforms suggested. The crucial aspects of the problem—the absence of accountability and the maintenance of the monopoly—would not have changed. Further, the underlying reason for reform was obscured by the hope of reform. According to Krause (1977), the physicians' grip on maintaining control of their work was weakening under pressure from new technology and new speciality occupations. The old craft-guild model was not up to controlling it all without some help from the state legislature. The help might follow the pattern of nurse-licensing laws in which the nurse's subservience to the physician would be written into the law (Krause, 1977), or new laws would be suggested that would institutionalize the physician as the manager of a system of health service delivery. In these ways, then, "reform" would aid the physician in adapting to the problem of role obsolescence. Still, licensing is the key utilized.

SELF-REGULATION BY PROFESSIONALS

American society has traditionally relied on professions to police themselves in the public interest. But the inadequacy of service to the public is a subject of increasing concern. Carlson (1975) notes that "Fragmentation, specialization, and a divergence between the goals of professionals and clients characterize all professional services today" (p. 46). In medicine, the high incidence of unnecessary and risky surgery, an overreadiness to prescribe inappropriate or dangerous medication, and the overuse of dangerous diagnostic measures tend to contribute to an escalation of iatrogenic (physician-caused) illness. In support, one report (Brown, 1978) included an elective surgery rate variation from seventy-four down to twenty-four per 10,000 in various regions in the state of Kansas; hospital infection rates varying from zero to twenty-four per 1,000; and justified hysterectomies varying from 20 to 80 percent among several hospitals. Scandals in Medicare, the willingness of lawyers to serve as "hired guns" for unethical or illegal client purposes, and the high reported incidence of faulty performance of common dental procedures all raise questions about self-policing. To what extent can self-regulation be effective? Are these isolated incidents or is the system unsound? What criteria should be met by a sound self-policing system?

Characteristics of an Effective Control System

The point of self-regulation is to limit the incidence of incompetent and unscrupulous service by professionals. How should we evaluate provisions for self-regulation by professionals? What criteria should be used to consider the adequacy of self-regulatory efforts? Donabedian's (1972) answer to these questions is most comprehensive. He discussed six attributes of an effective control system:

1. The system is ongoing to provide continued monitoring and reporting of data.
2. A corollary is that the system is regularly in place and organized so that its components are interdependent and mutually reinforcing rather than a slapped-together amalgam of random and ad hoc procedures.
3. The system monitors the outcomes of services as well as the processes.
4. When deviations from expected performance are detected, action is initiated that leads to investigation, prevention, and rehabilitation.
5. Consumers and related professionals are meaningfully involved in the control process along with representatives of the professionals being regulated.
6. Formal activities express and take their quality from the shared values and objectives of the informal organization of the professionals being regulated.

The idea of a system of control flies in the face of the professional value of autonomy. Daniels (1973) indicated:

There is really no reason to accept the contention that professional autonomy best meets the requirement for maintaining standards of professional service. For, whatever the rhetoric of professionalism, all the evidence seems to indicate that autonomy does not encourage the development of practical or workable systems of control. In medicine, for example, the ideal typical model of solo practice in a fee-for-service structure actively precludes the possibility of professional review. As a consequence, this profession with the greatest autonomy of any has a most fragmented system of professional control, while professions such as law and certified public accounting, which are not so independent and which must render account to extra-professional reviews, also possess more well-developed professional review systems. [pp. 54-55]

The research of Bucher and Stelling (1977) identified two themes in medical student socialization that undermine the effectiveness of colleague control. Medical trainees learn to discount the opinions of others, thus disavowing colleague control and affirming autonomous functioning. They learn about the inadequacy of the knowledge base in their field and they learn that most patients will improve regardless of what the physician does. It follows that they would reject the relevance of outcome measures and insist upon their own fallibility. Thus, physicians have little conceptual basis for faulting themselves or others. Physicians emphasize the process of their work performance as opposed to its outcome because they do not want to take responsibility for procedures they cannot predict, influence, or control. The lack of visibility of this process to anyone other than physicians and clients makes it difficult to determine standards by which colleagues could review the work of another physician. Bucher and Stelling did not fault professions for their inadequate knowledge bases, "But we do question the validity of the claim that professionals internalize high standards which result in self-monitoring and control" (p. 284).

Forms of Self-regulation

The types of control measures are described as the regulation of inputs, the monitoring of processes, and the evaluation of outputs. Output evaluation focuses on the results of treatment. There is a general absence of interest on the part of the professions or regulatory bodies in output measures. Input measures focus on the personnel offering service and the accreditation of their training and are discussed in this section under continuing education and recertification. Input measures also include licensing and certification activities of state licensing boards and professional associations. Process monitoring is concerned with how the service is offered and consists of various checks on the appropriateness of the service delivered. Informal disciplinary activities and peer reviews which tend to limit themselves to process monitoring are discussed in this section.

Discipline takes place in professional circles both formally and informally. Informal processes are both powerful and problematic. Because unethical, negligent, or exploitative behavior is often difficult to prove, and because the investigating professionals fear countersuit as a result of formal procedures, they may often rely on peer conversation. Since a good reputation is critical for success, and since a professional can be frozen out by the failure to receive referrals and consultation, a polite word in passing will sometimes curb questionable practice. If that is not effective, the pesonal boycott is the backup control measure used. A boycott, however, avoids dealing with the problem and gives no guidance or direction for a change in a provider's behavior. A problem with the informal process is that the same approach can also be used to control those professionals whose behavior is merely different or to smear those who threaten the professional status quo. In the absence of formal proceedings, it is difficult for professionals to restore their reputations, once damaged. The lack of accountability to the public, the infrequent and potentially capricious nature of the procedure, and the impossibility of measuring its extent or effect removes informal discipline from serious consideration as a way of encouraging or maintaining professional competence. Four other more formal means include continuing education, peer review, certification, and periodic recertification.

The provision of *continuing educational opportunities* and, particularly, the mandatory requirement of a set number of study hours of continuing education for recertification recognize that the knowledge on which professional practice is based becomes dated rapidly. While it seems reasonable to suppose that continuing education would have a positive impact on the practice of some providers, there remains a question whether continuing education should be mandated and whether it is, in fact, an effective corrective to incompetent practice. The move from voluntary to mandatory continuing education was stimulated by the belief that all professionals were not equally conscientious in keeping up with their fields. But to mandate something so loosely conceived as "continuing professional education" is an invitation to abuse. There is no assurance that professionals will take courses related to their practice. Even if they do, to expect an effect on performance assumes that professionals will know what they need to learn, will participate in such a way as to learn something, and then will be able to apply that learning to their practice, is tenuous. Since most courses focus on knowledge and since there is not necessarily a connection between knowledge and performance, it is unlikely that these courses would have an impact on practice. Shimberg (1977) and Carlson (1976) concluded after reviewing research that there were no demonstrated relationships between participation in continuing education programs and either job performance or measures of medical care outcomes. Williamson (1976) reported: "The track record regarding learning achievement for traditional continuing education courses is very low. Such courses may facilitate a momentary gain in knowledge, which often has short retention.

However, there is little or no evidence that these educational offerings change anyone's behavior" (p. 27).

Knox's review (1979) indicated continuing education programs can and do have impact, but many evaluators use expressions of participant satisfaction as their impact measure. There is, at best, only mixed evidence of a relationship between participant satisfaction and change in performance. One study reported by Carlson (1976) showed a positive relationship between *recent* medical school graduation and participation in continuing education. There seems reason to believe that those most in need of continuing education may be the least likely to receive it. The conclusion seems obvious that mandating continuing education has dubious value in providing consumers with protection against providers who fail to keep up to date.

Peer review is based on the belief that a knowledgeable third-party role, put in place to monitor the work of professionals, is an adequate deterrent to unethical, negligent, incompetent, and exploitative practice. Peer review is a retrospective process where data relating to performance, cost, or outcome may be monitored. Some forms of the peer review procedure utilized in the health professions follow.

Tissue committees of hospital physicians monitor the laboratory reports of tissue or organs removed in surgery to determine the necessity of operations according to the pathology of the tissue or organ. Other hospital-based review procedures are utilization review (which is concerned with the ongoing determination of the appropriateness of hospitalization, length of stays, and services rendered) and medical audit (which involves the review by an outside authority of a sample of patient hospital charts to determine whether care has been given according to accepted standards of practice). A medical audit may be done when there is controversy about the quality of medical care or as part of institutional accreditation.

Codes of ethics are formulated by professional associations to suit each profession's special requirements for practice. Standards are set for client protection (for example, confidentiality) as well as for competition among members (for example, advertising restraints). Depending on the size and extent of the organization, ethics committees may be formed on a national, statewide, regional, and even county level to receive complaints of ethics violations.

Grievance committees of professional associations are set up to respond to consumer complaints about the actions of their members. Complaints are usually about fees and obvious performance problems (for example, ill-fitting dentures).

Claims review concerns the monitoring by voluntary health insurance plans of physicians' charges and procedures to determine eligibility for payment, reasonableness of cost, and suitability of treatment.

Professional Standards Review Organizations (PSRO), authorized by

federal law in 1972, monitor the necessity and quality of impatient care provided to beneficiaries of federally funded programs (for example,
Medicare). Organized by areas containing a minimum of 300 physicians,
PSRO bring physicians together in an organization separate from the
medical society and the federal government to use peer review procedures.

It is typical in discussion by professionals of quality control measures to
cite a particular provision for such control (for example, a grievance committee) and assume that, because it is in place, it works. The failure to
separate potentiality from actuality thus tends to confuse discussion in this
area. There is no question that in the best of all possible worlds, *if*
professionals seriously decided that it was in their best interest to maintain
quality, peer review methods could significantly advance the achievement
of such purpose. A study conducted by *L'Office des Professions* in Quebec
(Bosk, 1977) revealed that some of the older professions had the power to
do so. They found that professional associations that were large, founded
before 1922, wealthy, made up of members engaged mainly in private practice with individual clients, and regulated by practice acts showed higher
levels of peer control than other professional associations. They did not
examine, however, whether this power was used in the public interest.

The critics of peer review point to an absence of will. An unusually candid
comment (Ingle, 1978) of a dentist attached to the National Academy of
Sciences who knew from personal experience the difference between "can"
and "will" was:

In 1954 I was the neophyte chairman of the Practice Plans Committee of the Seattle
District Dental Society. . . . Our first contract was with the International Long-
shoremen's and Warehousemen's Union-Pacific Maritime Association (ILWU-PMA)
to care for their children up to age 15. The late Goldie Krantz was the ILWU-PMA
negotiator. I'll never forget the rude shock when Mrs. Krantz asked, "How are you
going to police your members?" "Police," we answered, "what do you mean police?"
"Look," said Mrs. Krantz, "we're agreeing to pay out good money for dental care for
our kids. You're not naive enough to think we won't expect some strong measures
for controlling quality?" We were. . . . They wanted a high level committee written
into the contract—the best in the profession—to sit in judgment of their peers; and if
the quality of a dentist's treatment was found wanting, he was to be dropped from
the program. "We don't intend to haggle over fees," the Union said, "so in turn, we
expect quality care for our money." And quality they got, though more than a few
dentists were censured and/or dropped from the panel. (pp. vii-viii]

PSRO, the most comprehensive cooperation between a profession and
the federal government to attempt to achieve effective peer review, works
when properly applied. According to Brown (1978) hospital stays were
reduced by 20 percent in one PSRO; a 20 percent reduction of the need for
surgery after a second opinion was given occurred in another; an increase
was noted in the effectiveness of disease pathology diagnosis related to

appendicitis from 18 to 55 percent after a medical audit; and a decline in antibiotic use from 60 to 30 percent occurred in another.

Criticism of peer review generally suggests that it maintains the autonomy of professionals while giving the appearance that behavior injurious to the public is being eliminated. In general, Donabedian's (1972) criteria are not fulfilled. The voluntary involvement of professionals, the advisory nature of most reports, and the general lack of agreement on standards testify to sporadic monitoring and ad hoc procedures. Professionals generally are reluctant to comment on each other's practice. Their failure to do so voluntarily has caused fifteen states to require individual physicians to report instances of other physicians' abuse of patients; eight states require medical societies to do so. Medical peer review processes focus on business concerns of professionals, fraud, and cost to the public indicating the avoidance of concern for the quality of care or outcomes. Referring to the dual function of PSRO, utilization, and quality control, Somers and Somers (1977) concluded, "As long as the costs of Medicaid and Medicare continue their astronomical rise, it is likely that the government will increasingly stress the utilization aspects" (p. 277).

Peer review responds to complaints and when there is action it is punitive in orientation, rarely concerned with prevention or effective rehabilitation. When public members or related professionals are included in review processes, they are usually token, and they are easily co-opted. The substantial amount of information developed by PSRO is not shared with the public, so there is very little external influence. In fact, Annas (1976) alleged that physicians and hospitals would not cooperate voluntarily with PSRO if the data were to be made public. The difficulty consumers have in finding out to whom to complain and in making complaints testifies to the low esteem in which peer review is held in professional circles. Judith Rosner (1979) reported on structured interviews with eighty-nine Fort Worth, Texas, dentists. She found that 51 percent judged peer review as not being useful. Claiming differences of opinion among dentists, dislike of criticizing one another, or unfamiliarity with conditions of work, dentists expressed their reluctance to exert influence on one another. This triumph of form over substance in peer review results from the need to maintain the reputation of the profession and by so doing ward off public scrutiny that might limit autonomy and freedom from lay control. Ethics committees give the appearance of attention to matters of standards and morals, but they rarely act and, when they do, the action tends to be pallid. But by giving the appearance of concern they have warded off more stringent public regulation of professionals. According to Lieberman (1970), the theory of discipline followed by professionals distinguishes between public and private behavior. Discipline was only for public unorthodoxy, he asserted. Therefore, when the public is ignorant of the misdeeds of a professional, there is no need to act, since a review would call attention to it. It followed, in this reasoning, that there was no reason to disbar or eject a member permanently as the public was likely to forget.

Certification refers to individual credentialing by professional associations and has become an important means of regulating entry into the professions and to specializations within professions. In medicine the process of credentialing specialists began in 1916 with the establishment of the American Board of Opthalmology. Presently there are twenty-three certifying agencies in medicine. The American Board of Examiners in Professional Psychology (ABEPP) fulfills a similar function for psychologists. Health service credentialing is also done by the Board of Registry of Medical Technologists of the American Society of Clinical Pathologists, the American Registry of Inhalation Therapists, the American Registry of Radiological Technologists, the American Occupational Therapy Association, the National Environmental Health Association, and the American Medical Record Association. Certification, as distinct from licensure, is under the direct control of professions and is national in scope, so with regard to their certification the professions do not have to deal with fifty-one separate jurisdictions. As a result, members can be professionally mobile across state lines. Certification provides visibility and increased respectability for dietitians and mental health counselors, for example, despite the fact that only one state licenses mental health counselors and two states license dietitians. In other cases, professional certification has become the basis for an indirect form of licensing. The use of certified personnel may be mandated by state or federal law and third-party insurance carriers for reimbursement for services.

Periodic *recertification* and relicensure on the basis of continuing education or examination was introduced in 1967 by the National Advisory Commission on Health Manpower (Welch, 1973). It was not until the 1970s that some medical specialty boards began issuing certificates with expiration dates. The previous assumption was that certificates issued without expiration dates were valid until the death of the recipient. Although all twenty-three medical specialty boards currently endorse the concept of periodic recertification, there is a great deal of variation in implementation. The leader in the field is the American Board of Family Practice. When it was established in 1969, it required mandatory recertification after six years of practice with reexamination essential for continued certification. The American College of Physicians introduced voluntary self-assessment examinations in 1967. The American Board of Surgery has required recertification for those receiving certification after 1975, but reexamination is voluntary. The American Board of Internal Medicine's reexamination program is entirely voluntary. Other boards use participation in continuing education, self-assessment examinations, or practice audits as criteria for recertification.

Recertification was suggested as early as 1940, but it took thirty years to become a viable concept, as professionals generally fear reevaluation of their credentials. The recommendations of the American Board of Medical Specialties (ABMS), though endorsing recertification, warned specialty boards not to rescind certificates unless a date of expiration was a condition of the original certification, thus grandfathering the great majority of medical specialists, regardless of their real competence. Genuine meaning to the specialty identification is further compromised by the fact that physicians may, with the blessing of the American Medical Association, simply proclaim themselves to be specialists *without* meeting specialty board requirements.

The value of the certification procedure in medicine has been questioned by Williamson (1976). He had a difficult time "finding evidence of the relation of certification results to actual clinical performance . . ." (p. 20). The evidence he did find indicated that "certification results, whether measured by professional undergraduate grades or medical specialty certification examinations, seem to have very little relationship to quality of subsequent professional performance" (p. 25). He recommended that examination content be related to the heterogeneous range of problems presented by patients and that the methods used to determine competence cover a broader range of actual performance by physicians, the implication being that certification methods had a poor record on both counts.

Recertification as practiced by the American Board of Family Practice comes closest to meeting Donabedian's (1972) criteria by requiring a periodic examination with performance features. Other boards, by avoiding performance examinations or by making the entire process voluntary, bow to the preferences of physicians over the needs of the public, indicating the triumph in self-regulation of form over substance. The "field-force" analysis shown in table 5.1 (drawn from an article by two members of the National Board of Medical Examiners) reveals pressure toward recertification to be largely external to the professions and extensive foot-dragging from within the profession.

Only if mandatory recertification is based on performance evaluation, and if other agencies and institutions (for example, hospitals, health insurance, and governments, in the case of medicine) level appropriate economic sanctions to require that standards be met, can we regard recertification as an acceptable form of self-regulation.

ALTERNATIVES TO THE GUILD MODEL

Engel and Hall (1973) pointed out that the common view of professions rested on "a conception of professional work as typically entrepreneurial and individualistic" (p. 76). They noted changes that were altering working patterns in the professions so that more professionals are either working in bureaucracies or finding their work situations becoming more bureaucratically organized. Sophistication in technology and greater specialization estab-

TABLE 5.1 Field-Force Diagram

Driving Forces toward Recertification	Restraining Forces on Recertification
Specialty boards acknowledged accountability and perceived logic of recertification (ABMS)	Reluctance of physicians to accept change because of challenge to status
Impending federal or state requirements	Professional concern over compulsion and government control
Possible hospital and institutional requirements	Lack of fully defined criteria of competence in specialties
Malpractice crisis	No fully developed validated profiling system for physicians
Private third-party carriers requirements	Difficulty in setting standard of performance
Corporations, labor unions, and other large purchasers	Need for funding of recertification implementation
Specialty societies	Problem of large group of physicians not certified at all
CCME[1]-LCGME[2] and LCCME[3]	No strategy for coping with physicians who fail
Physicians's desire for excellence and recognition	Demand on physician's time for continuing medical education and recertification
Forces from "state of the art" methodology becoming available for evaluation	Low priority of recertification among health care needs
Rising consumer awareness through public education	Lack of availability of established process and outcome measures
Peer review—foundations, PSRO, and so on	Present questions on relevance and validity of competence measures
Internal Revenue Service	Potential negative impact on size of manpower pool

Source: Robert A. Chase and Frederic D. Burg, Reexamination/Recertification, *Archives of Surgery,* 1977, 112(1), 22. Copyright 1977, American Medical Association.

[1]Coordinating Council on Medical Education (CCME).
[2]Liaison Committee on Graduate Medical Education (LCGME).
[3]Liaison Committee on Continuing Medical Education (LCCME).

lished, according to Engel and Hall, "a need for both a greater division of labor and teams of hierarchically organized work groups functioning within and across professional lines" (p. 77). The pressure in bureaucracies to make the professional indistinguishable from the bureaucrat is resisted by professional norms which in turn alter bureaucratic norms, but in the end the professional work pattern has changed. Engel and Hall (1973) summarized and compared these changes in table 5.2.

The client lost some confidentiality and personalization of service in exchange for multiple relationships with more highly trained specialists in an organizational setting that took more responsibility for quality control. In exchange for freedom from daily economic pressures, professionals permitted increased visibility of their performance. This visibility allowed for greater peer and public evaluation. It is expected that the effect of greater visibility would be better quality control.

Considering these changes, the need for autonomy and self-regulation is no longer apparent. Autonomy and self-regulation are justified mainly for nonbureaucratic professionals because outsiders lack the knowledge and ability to observe and judge the performance of professionals. Knowledge is becoming available and even standardized so that paraprofessionals may perform duties previously considered solely professional duties. Observation by peers, by professionals from other occupations, and by the public is increasingly possible.

This bureaucratization of the professions has created work patterns much like those of the scientist. Scientists share many characteristics with licensed professionals (for example, calling, knowledge, association, and altruism), but because the norms of science dictate against the monopoly of knowledge, because scientists tend to work for institutions, and because as scientists they do not deliver direct services to individuals or groups, scientific practice has not required the attribute of autonomy. This suggests that the scientist model may be an alternative one for the professions. Goode (1960) compared the two models explaining, "Throughout Western history, most professionals have been bureaucrats: the military officer, the clergyman, the university professor, most engineers and architects, and much earlier both the lawyer and the physician" (p. 906). He went on to say that a new development is the extensive division of labor which now permits the

employment of the scientist essentially for his skill in science. The science, not the bureaucracy, defines employment standards, and because the work is largely science, not art, it can be evaluated with some precision. Competence can be tested, and thus there is less need for either certification or licensure, or guild protection. Professional monopoly of a *scientific* field seems impossible or absurd. [p. 906]

Hughes (1965) noted a countervailing tendency toward a guild model for scientists. He distinguished between guild professions, such as medicine and

TABLE 5.2 Evolving Professional Characteristics

Traditional Characteristics	Modified Characteristics
1. Isolated individual provides services	Teams provide service
2. Knowledge from a single discipline typically utilized	Knowledge from diverse fields typically utilized
3. Remuneration predominantly fee-for-service	Remuneration predominantly by salary
4. Altruism: Selfless service limited by entrepreneurialism	Altruism: Increased opportunity for selfless service
5. Restricted colleague evaluation of product	Increased opportunity for colleague evaluation of product
6. Privacy in client-professional relationship	Decreased privacy in client-professional relationship

Source: Reprinted from Gloria V. Engel and Richard H. Hall, "The Growing Industrialization of the Professions," p. 85, in Eliot Freidson, ed., *The Professions and Their Prospects* © 1973 by Sage Publications, Inc., with permission.

engineering, that "pursue knowledge to improve practice" and the scientific models, such as archeology and physics, that are "professions by accident . . . where the practices are merely the means to increasing knowledge" (p. 6). In some fields there is a tendency for the "distinction to disappear and for the learned societies to become professional guilds concerned with problems of practice, employment, licensing and distribution of their service" (p. 7).

Another alternative offers a radical proposal that reveals by contrast the nature of professionalism. Sarason and Lorentz (1979) were very critical of professionalism, describing it as "quintessentially a quest for personal and social worth" (p. 112). They described professional preciousness (acts that manifest disdain for nonprofessionals) and professional imperialism (acts that increase a profession's monopoly of practice) as social diseases which require that problems be defined and solved in such ways as to necessitate the services of professionals. This behavior created "a gulf between the professions and the public, and among the professions . . . [which is] a stance that downgrades two-way exchanges of any kind and elevates *noblesse oblige* as a basis for interaction: Resources flow in one direction because the recipient is seen as devoid of relevant resources" (p. 113). Sarason and Lorentz (1979) suggested the resource exchange network as a model for knowledge utilization that contrasts with the professional model of knowledge utilization. They based the model on three assumptions.

1. Those affected by the decision of others need to be involved in the decision making in some nonritualistic way.
2. Individual lives and the larger society are too important to be left to the judgment of professionals.
3. The process by which professionals are trained "always results in attitudes that make it extremely uncomfortable for the professional (and often impossible) to share decision making with others affected by his or her decisions" (p. 115).

Resource exchange networks are exemplified by self-help groups. The hostility self-help groups encounter from professionals is understandable since they offer a clear alternative to professional knowledge exchange. Their characteristics offer a contrast to professional-client interaction.

1. There are no second-class citizens, all members have the same rights and obligations and participate voluntarily.
2. Resource networks permit learning opportunities unrestrained by conventional credentialing criteria and limited only by the knowledge, interests, skills, and talents of their members.
3. Resource networks are open to the entry of new members, as well as to diverse persons, diversity being an antidote to parochialism.
4. Resource networks have hierarchies of talent but these hierarchies are flexible, permitting shifts depending on needs, topics, or issues.
5. Resource networks appear to be unstable because they are functional systems which deal with matters of actual or potential need, adopting new missions and objectives as necessary.

Sarason and Lorentz (1979) were critical of professionalism because professional status and power were seen as obstacles to resource utilization by society at a time when society needed more resources. Because of their status and power, professionals cannot be treated like anyone else. Professions tend to limit resources and focus on deficits rather than strengths at a time when what is needed is a radical redefinition of human resources that emphasizes what people can do about personal and social problems rather than what they cannot do. They were not naive, however, as they recognized that professionalism had strong, societal support. After all, "It is not technical need that leads to turfdom and *noblesse oblige* but fear, greed, and insecurity" and it is that aspect of "the culture that made for a positive response to the cult of professionalism" (pp. 128-29). Perhaps the negative response in the last decade, the process by which exclusiveness breeds obsolescence, the awareness of the problems associated with professionalism, and the social changes involved in the bureaucratization of the professions are all indicative of some basic changes in the need for the "quick fix" of professionalism and will force continuing alterations in the models a society develops for knowledge utilization.

6

LICENSING BOARDS AND THE REGULATORY PROCESS

The authority for interpreting and implementing state law regarding professional licensure in the United States over the last century has been given to a state administrative entity often referred to as a "board." These boards have several forms, as indicated in table 6.1. Some states have separate, autonomous boards for particular professions, while others bring together some or all functions in centralized agencies for one, several or a variety of professions. Following the Roederer and Shimberg (1980) model used in table 6.1, the transition from autonomous board to centralized agency is characterized first by the takeover of housekeeping functions; second, such control functions as budget, staff, and investigation are transferred to the central agency; third, policy determination and implementation are reviewed by the central agency; and finally, these latter policy functions are assumed by the central agency. Seventeen states reported that more than one model prevailed, with many combining fully autonomous models with minor (models A and B) or moderate limits (models A and C). Though there has been growth in the number of boards subsumed by central agencies for part or all of their functions, in forty-four states boards operate with a minimum of external review or control. The autonomous licensing board is currently alive and well.

This pattern of decentralized authority for regulation is consistent with the development of governmental structures in the United States, particularly in those areas traditionally covered by the State's police powers to guarantee the welfare of each citizen. Though this authority had been held at one time by educational institutions and professional organizations, in the United States there has been resistance to any effort to nationalize what has become a highly decentralized and differentiated system. Roemer's (1973) review of legal systems in seven foreign countries revealed a central governmental or quasi-governmental authority licensing physicians in Japan, Sweden, Columbia, the United Kingdom, and France. A nominal

TABLE 6.1 Models of Organization for State Occupational Licensing Boards in the United States

Description	Model A	Model B	Model C	Model D	Model E
Autonomy	*Full*	*Minor Limits*	*Moderate Limits*	*Limited Autonomy*	*Not Autonomous*
ACTIVITIES:					
1. Decide about office location, purchasing, and procedures	Board	Central Agency	Central Agency	Central Agency	Central Agency
2. Collects fees and handles financial records	Board	Central Agency	Central Agency	Central Agency	Central Agency
3. Handles applications	Board	Central Agency	Central Agency	Central Agency	Central Agency
4. Responds to inquiries	Board	Central Agency	Central Agency	Central Agency	Central Agency
5. Issues licenses and renewals	Board	Central Agency	Central Agency	Central Agency	Central Agency
6. Hires staff	Board	Board	Central Agency	Central Agency	Central Agency
7. Receives and investigates complaints	Board	Board	Central Agency	Central Agency	Central Agency

Table 6.1—(continued)

Description	Model A	Model B	Model C	Model D	Model E
Autonomy	*Full*	*Minor Limits*	*Moderate Limits*	*Limited Autonomy*	*Not Autonomous*
ACTIVITIES:					
8. Budgetary control	Board	Board	Central Agency	Central Agency	Central Agency
9. Disciplines licensees	Board	Board	Board	Board*	Central Agency†
10. Responsible for entry examination procedures	Board	Board	Board	Board*	Central Agency†
11. Sets qualifications	Board	Board	Board	Board*	Central Agency†
12. Decides who is qualified	Board	Board	Board	Board*	Central Agency†
13. Sets standards for practice	Board	Board	Board	Board*	Central Agency†
Number of states (predominant model)	19	7	18	4	2

Source: Doug Roederer and Benjamin Shimberg, *Occupational Licensing: Centralizing State Licensure Functions* (Lexington, Ky.: Council of State Governments, 1980), p. 4.
*Board actions are reviewed by central agency.
†Where boards exist, they are advisory.

authority was held by states or provinces in West Germany and Poland, but effective policy control was centered in the national government. Roemer also found that a much greater reliance was placed on the university systems in these countries to make the determination of competence.

CHARACTERISTICS

The licensing board is an administrative unit that receives power from a state's legislature to permit or to regulate both occupational activities and the use of occupational titles. The legislative act usually involves the creation of a board as an administrative agency and the determination of its authority and composition. Boards are a part of the executive branch of state government but are somewhat unique since they also fulfill legislative and judicial functions. The legislative function refers to rule-making authority, which has the force of law. Judicial authority refers to judgments relative to denial, suspension, or revocation of licenses or to the discipline of licensees. A great deal more will be said about these functions in a later section of this chapter. Reviewed before that will be the role of administrative process in the operation of the licensing board, the specific powers and duties assigned to licensing boards, and the composition of these boards.

Licensing boards are administrative arms of state government and as such are usually guided by an administrative procedures act. These acts set the requirements for the legislative function of rule making. Administrative procedures acts also determine the limits of agency authority with regard to disciplinary proceedings and describe appeal procedures. This standardization of procedure in a variety of agencies is seen as a greater safeguard to the rights of individuals. The probability is reduced of differing, perhaps capricious, standards were agencies permitted to set up their own procedures. These acts usually focus primary jurisdiction in particular agencies and require appeals to be reviewed by agencies before being taken to a court to be heard (Waddle, 1979).

The powers and duties assigned to licensing boards relate to the control of entrance into the practice of a profession and the enforcement of standards of practice among those licensed. In the pursuit of these objectives licensing boards will usually act in the following ways:

1. Receive and examine the credentials of applicants to determine if they meet statutory and administrative requirements.
2. Decide what training programs meet the requirements for preparing applicants to meet credentialing standards.
3. Prepare, administer, and grade competency assessments; determining those who meet and those who fail to meet the criterion.
4. Grant licenses to persons who meet the competency criteria or to those from other states who meet the reciprocity criteria.

5. Establish standards of practice, investigate violations, conduct hearings, pass judgment on the facts, and warn, suspend, revoke, and reinstate a license or otherwise penalize a licensee.

6. Collect fees and fines and control and disburse funds at their disposal.

The people who sit on licensing boards and the ways they became board members have undergone some changes since the early licensing boards. Many of the early licensing laws required that board members be elected by the members of the professional associations they were to regulate. Those elected were not to be reviewed by any governmental authority. Though this system was superseded by systems in which state governors chose board members from lists supplied by professional associations, Waddle (1979) pointed to the Oklahoma Dental Practice Act as one where board members were still elected by members of a professional association. The system of selecting board members from association lists has mostly given way to systems where these groups are allowed to give input and where appointing officials can, but need not, consider that input. Tochen's (1978) study of six occupations indicated that of 298 boards, 54 required that members be appointed from lists prepared by licensed professionals or by professional associations.

Licensing laws usually indicate the number and composition of the board. They may stipulate the inclusion of consumer or public representatives, active practitioners, members of related occupations, and those who teach in the educational programs of the occupation. Depending on the profession, boards may be composed of members of the profession only, members of related professions only, or a mixture of the two. Dental hygienists, for example, are licensed by dental boards that include no hygienists, while veterinarians are licensed by boards that with few exceptions are composed entirely of veterinarians.

Hogan (1979b) studied the composition of state psychology boards. The average board size was five or six, while the range varied from three to twelve. Only 10 percent of psychology board members were representatives of the public. For the most part board members' qualifications required that they be licensed psychologists with up to five years' experience as practicing psychologists. They were generally selected by governors from lists supplied by state psychological associations not because the governors were required to appoint those preferred by the associations but generally because of lobbying efforts by associations. The term of office for psychology board members was usually three to five years with about half the states limiting the number of consecutive terms a board member may serve to one or two. Board members may be removed from office either by the board itself in some states or the governor in others. Neglect of duty, incompetence, and misconduct are common grounds for removal. Board members so charged have the right to a notice and a hearing.

Shimberg (1979) revealed some of the problems and confusion surrounding the practice of including public members on boards. The hope has been expressed that public members would be "lobbyists for the people" who would ensure that the views of the public would gain a hearing during board discussions. The reality is that governors tend to see these positions as part of their patronage and fill the vacancies without regard to these expectations. Shimberg (1979) concluded that the public member approach has been unsuccessful because of the belief "that anyone who was not a member of the regulated occupation was eligible to be a public member" (p. 11). Public members without special interests or qualifications soon discover the meetings to be dull, the language confusing, the interests at stake submerged, and the prestige and prerogatives to be minimal. If they continue to attend meetings their confusion is often clarified by well-meaning professionals, thus co-opting the special role the public member was to play. Shimberg contrasted professional and public members on variables relating to motivation and satisfaction as indicated in table 6.2 and suggested the appropriate question was not, why are public members so ineffectual? But how do they accomplish anything at all?

Gilb (1966) discussed the power professional associations have over licensing boards as deriving from direct or indirect involvement in appointments. She described the procedure of a particular governor, who inquired into the professional background of each appointee; the purpose being the balancing of factions. This tended to exclude new and not-quite-legitimized elements of the professions and served to ensure that "no one was appointed to whom the associations objected" (p. 196).

Some boards are financed solely by the fees of licensees while others receive general revenue funds from the State. Fees vary greatly. Whitesel (1977) pointed out that the range in Wisconsin was from no charge for certified building inspectors to $750 per year for licensed liquor manufacturers. Shimberg (1979) showed that some boards have heavy responsibilities but insufficient resources because some states' legislatures divert fees income to other purposes. Tochen's (1978) study of the licensing boards for veterinarians, optometrists, barbers, funeral directors or embalmers, accountants, and pharmacists showed boards in twenty-three states receiving all their funds from licensing or other fees, but five were required to deposit a small percentage of funds in the state's general fund. In sixteen states boards were financed totally from state general funds. In eleven states there is a combination of these two methods of financing. On the other hand, in psychology, Hogan (1979b) found all the state boards to be self-sustaining. The self-sustaining approach has been criticized as placing the board in a dependent position financially on those it must regulate, thus perverting the regulatory process into a dues-paying club which only does what the members are willing to pay for. But a more immediate problem is that fees are an insufficient basis for funding vigorous

TABLE 6.2 **Contrast between Professional and Public Members on Variables Associated with Motivations and Satisfactions of Licensing Board Members**

Professional Members	Factor	Public Members
Very concerned	**Peer group**	None
Great deal	**Prestige**	Little
Vital	**Interest in professional issues**	Not involved
Extension of professional life, willing to devote substantial time	**Time**	Adverse financial impact, unwilling to devote a great deal of time
Experienced as a licensee	**Familiarity with licensing process**	Ordinarily little
Professional association has data, personnel, organization	**Availability of independent, supportive resources**	Usually none

Source: Benjamin Shimberg, "Recruiting and Selecting Members for Occupational Licensing Boards," Remarks before Advisory Committee Appointed by Governor Graham to Recommend Individuals for Board Membership (Tallahassee, Fla.: April 11, 1979), pp. 12-13.

investigation and enforcement procedures. Boards that do not pursue investigation and enforcement often wind up with the opposite problem of having large surpluses, having taken in more money in fees and fines than they have spent in regulation. Tochen (1978) found one state (South Dakota) that had a unique way of disposing of its surplus. After funds were set aside to run the optometric board for the year, the remaining balance was transferred to the Optometric Association for its own uses and purposes.

Accountability requirements vary. Of the 298 boards that Tochen (1978) studied, 25 were not required to keep minutes of their meetings and 142 were not required to file annual or biannual reports. Even in those states that required meetings and reports, it was often difficult to determine the extent to which boards were complying with the law, there being few if any sanctions to use against noncomplying boards. No state required the detailed accounting of finances and activities that Tochen (1978) believed essential, indicating information about the disposition of license applications and complaints. Tochen did find that all states had open-meeting laws, though the matter of notifying the public of a meeting to be held is often handled so poorly that many boards have no public attendance at their meetings. The failure to publish notices in community newspapers causes the public to be unaware of meetings while short notification (for example, one day) causes inconvenience.

Boards have operated with generally little legislative oversight. The exception, sunset review, will be discussed at the conclusion of this chapter. One study (Virginia, 1982) reported recently on a review of nine licensing boards in Virginia. Six of the nine had promulgated regulations without statutory authority. More than one-quarter of these boards' standards regarding practice and entry were judged to be questionable or unnecessary. Complaint handling came in for special criticism. The report noted that almost 1,000 complaints had been filed with Better Business Bureau or consumer affairs offices rather than the appropriate board. Where complaints did reach the boards, one-half of the reviews were completed before the investigations were finished and many were closed without disciplinary action being taken or a resolution being achieved about the consumer's grievance. Earlier, in California, Summerfield (1978) reported on the processing time for complaints to California's Psychology Examining Committee (table 6.3), revealing a similar insensitivity to consumer reactions.

TABLE 6.3 Processing Time for Complaints* to California's Psychology Examining Committee, according to Source

Source	Average Number of Days	Standard Deviation (Days)	N (Cases)
Patients	454	555	48
Professional community	252	244	29
State agencies	224	161	43

Source: H. L. Summerfield, *Review of Psychology Examining Committee and State Board of Behavioral Science Examiners: A Report of the Regulatory Review Task Force* (State of California, Department of Consumer Affairs, 1978), p. I-21.

*Includes cases open as of March 25, 1978. Does not include cases rejected prior to investigation.

FUNCTIONS OF BOARDS

This section will focus on the description of specific board functions: rule making, entry restriction, and standards maintenance. The effectiveness of boards in fulfilling these functions is reviewed in chapter 8.

Rule making underlies the entire operation of the licensing board. The board is created to place the authority for translating every restrictions and standards enforcement in particular administrative units. Though statutes describe general expectations for implementation, it is up to the board to make the expectations operational through specific requirements and procedures. Generally the boards have wide latitude in determining standards, in deciding the criteria for standards enforcement, in defining unprofessional conduct, in interpreting eligibility requirements, in preparing and grading competency assessment, and in determining what training is acceptable for their applicants. Courts normally uphold the actions of boards as long as they act in conformity with the enabling legislation. Though there are stated limits on the authority of boards to act (for example, no arbitrary action, no action that deprives persons of their constitutional rights), the interpretation of these limits is varied and the review of board action is minimal and at best episodic. The need to familiarize board members with the basic requirements of admnistrative and constitutional law was recognized recently by the National Association of Attorneys General which published in 1978 its *Rulemaking Manual for Occupational Licensing Boards*. The act of rule making ordinarily places an administrative unit in a powerful position but when it is combined with an absence of review and of checks and balances because legislative, executive, and judicial functions are combined in one unit, we can see with Shimberg (1979) that "There can be little doubt that what boards do can have profound implications for those who wish to practice a trade or profession as well as those who use the services of those licensed by the board" (p. 5).

Setting eligibility standards is an entry restriction function of boards. The determination is made about which applicants are to be permitted to demonstrate their competency. Personal characteristics such as age, residency, citizenship, and "moral character" are usually cited as entry criteria. In some states a minimum age will be specified for some occupations but not for others. In Wisconsin you must be aged twenty-three to become a certified public accountant but there is no stated minimum age for dentists, chiropractors, or registered nurses. About half of the licensed occupations in California specify age twenty-one as a minimum.

State residency and U.S. citizenship is specified in some states. Hogan (1979b) reported that sixteen states required psychologists to be U.S. citizens or to have declared their intent to become a citizen, while ten states required psychologists to be state residents. Citizenship requirements are under increasing attack and are considered to have dubious legality. Interpretations of U.S. Supreme Court decisions in *McLaughlin* v. *Florida* (1964) and *Sugarman* v. *Dugall* (1973) suggest that statutory citizenship requirements deprive resident aliens from benefits mandated by the Fourteenth Amendment, according to Whitesel (1977).

Good moral character is rarely defined positively. If it is defined it is likely to be defined negatively so as to exclude applicants who have been convicted of a felony, particular misdemeanors, or crimes involving moral turpitude. Applicants are often required to submit affidavits or testimonials that they are of "good moral character." Though in some cases the motive for this restriction is to bar persons who might likely profit by opportunities for dishonest gain, there are many occupations in which opportunities for dishonest gain are quite limited yet they have these restrictions. Public image is seen as the real motive in these cases. California has proscribed boards from barring entry on the basis of a past crime unless it can be demonstrated that the crime is work related (Haberfield et al., 1978). In a few cases, boards impose bonding requirements or proof of financial assets (for example, contractors) as a way of protecting the public against fraud or misrepresentation.

Educational and experience requirements are usually included as part of the entry restriction function of boards. They are usually stated in terms of minimal years of schooling and experience. The type of training (for example, approved schools) and the nature of the supervision of experience may be specified as well. Lack of expertise and limitations on personnel and funds often mean that the boards do not usually make their own determination but rather rely on lists of accredited schools approved by the professional association. Professional associations have not always used these powers in the best interests of the public. Noted previously was the decline of medical school enrollments following the Flexner report and their failure to keep pace with a growing population. Haberfield et al. (1978) asserted that the American Medical Association used its accrediting power granted by state licensing boards to pressure schools to restrict admissions. Joy (1977) reported that in Michigan in 1910 there was one registered optometrist for every 3,722 persons; the ratio in 1970 was one to 9,431. There was a flurry of interest in the early 1970s to substitute proficiency testing of skills in place of educational and experience requirements. Professional associations have opposed such changes and their implementation has been minimal (Waddle, 1979). Apprenticeship requirements may specify a number of years of experience in the office of a licensed practitioner. In this case the entry to a field is determined by the extent to which private practitioners are willing to employ prospective applicants for the prescribed period.

Assessment of competency usually involves a written examination covering the content of preparatory training and may involve oral and practical application examinations. The exams may be prepared and administered locally by the boards themselves or, increasingly, may be handled on a national level by a testing service or professional association (Shimberg, 1981). There is a great deal of variety in the quality of these examinations with many local exams not meeting well-recognized reliability and validity requirements and ignoring the equal employment opportunity guidelines that they be based on a task analysis of the profession (Whitesel, 1977). Assessment of competency is discussed further in chapter 7. The purpose of examinations is supposed to be an estimation of the fitness of the

applicant to fulfill the obligations of professional practice consistent with
the requirements of public welfare. The manner in which boards fulfill this
charge may affect the opportunity that applicants have to demonstrate their
fitness. Boards set fees for examinations and some may be high enough to
discourage applications. The frequency with which the examinations are
offered and the accessibility of the sites where they take place may inhibit
some applicants. Delay in reporting the results can be an interference in
initiating practice, thus discouraging some. Setting or adjusting the pass-fail
standard has a direct impact on entry. Finally, the right to appeal the
board's decision may not be easily available so that applicants can be
discouraged from learning how they might be more successful at a later
time. Waddle (1979) questioned whether the following procedures were in
place to aid unsuccessful candidates:

Were standards set for the examination and its evaluation?
Were the standards applied the same for all examinees?
Were there objective criteria for evaluation?
Is the record available for the grades and for the method of grading?
Are you prepared to allow the unsuccessful examinee to review the examination
questions and answers used in grading the particular examination? [p. 142]

The extreme variety in the eligibility standards approved by fifty state
boards has necessitated the development of procedures that either facilitate
or inhibit the transfer of professionals from one state to another. Known as
reciprocity, it is a procedure that either grants a license to a practitioner
from a state that has equivalent eligibility and examination standards or
permits applicants to sit for the examination if they come from states that
have lower standards. Failure to meet age, citizenship, or residency
requirements may block eligibility, or a score on a national exam lower
than a state's cutoff score may require a probationer to retake the exam.
There is a great deal of variety from state to state and from occupation to
occupation concerning the ease or difficulty in obtaining reciprocity. The
consequences of reciprocity standards are discussed in chapter 8. The use of
national examinations as a substitute for local examinations has been an
option for some occupations to reduce the difficulty practitioners have in
moving from one state to another.

In the area of standards maintenance, boards have three functions:
discipline, competency maintenance, and competition restraints. Enforcement of the rules and regulations governing practice generally takes the
form of receiving complaints, performing investigations, hearing evidence,
judging the licensee, and revoking or suspending licenses or issuing repri-
mands. In some instances state law would require certain concerns (for
example, fraud) to be referred to local or state law enforcement authorities.
The purpose of the disciplinary role is to ensure that practitioners continue
to serve the public in a safe and competent manner. How effectively licensing boards discharge this function depends on whether enabling statutes

contain the necessary grounds on which to base disciplinary actions and the extent of vigorous handling of consumer complaints and investigations. Consumer groups have added a third condition that the laws should provide complainants with a specific way by which they might recoup any losses sustained as the result of unsafe or incompetent treatment. Lack of board jurisdiction, vaguely written grounds, poor complaint handling, rare investigations on matters of competence, and poor funding bases for disciplinary activity are some of the criticisms of the role of licensing boards. Licensing boards have rather broad discretion in these matters and have tended to see the license as a property right; thus they have been reluctant to act as often or as vigorously as their critics have desired. The problem is dealt with further in chapter 8.

Boards prescribe standards of conduct presumably as a guide to rendering safe and ethical services. Ordinarily, however, these rules only restrain competition among professionals. Some boards have set minimum price schedules, while others limit the number of branch offices, soliciting, including the use of "steerers" to direct trade, and "no raiding" pacts (Haberfield et al., 1978). The primary form of such regulation, however, is restriction on the time, place, and manner of advertising. Tochen's (1978) survey found that eighteen states limited veterinarians from advertising prices or services, while only one state expressly permitted it under certain circumstances. Accountants are not directly permitted to advertise in any state and are prohibited from advertising in forty-two states. Overcast et al. (1982) indicated that the states have been relatively free of antitrust scrutiny, which the Federal Trade Commission and the Department of Justice have applied to the professions, but these regulations must clearly be state policy and actively supervised by the state. Anticompetitive standards of conduct must be differentiated from policies of the regulated occupations.

Maintaining continuing competence has recently meant the mandating of continuing education. In 1967 the National Advisory Commission on Health Manpower recommended the updating of qualifications through continuing education. The hope was that practitioners would develop understanding of new knowledge and new skill so as to sustain their competence. Relicensure of practitioners depends on the completion of a specified number of hours of advanced training. By requiring continuing education, states have given up on policies based on the belief that practitioners would voluntarily keep up with the knowledge explosion. The limitations of this approach are discussed in chapters 5 and 8. An alternative approach to maintaining competence is the periodic reexamination of competence. Opposed by most professionals, periodic reexamination has not been adopted by any licensing board.

THE REGULATORY PROCESS

The problem of regulation is the difference between what is espoused as its purpose and what it actually accomplishes. The effects of what has been done have raised questions about the purposes. Gellhorn's (1976) analysis was that "a well-knit special interest group is likely to prevail over an amorphous 'public' whose members are dispersed and, as individuals, are not in sharp conflict with the organized interest" (p. 16). Some of the consequences of this imbalance of interest follow.

Occupational licensing has typically brought higher status for the producer of services at the price of higher costs to the consumer; it has reduced competition; it has narrowed opportunity for aspiring youth by increasing the costs of entry into a desired occupational career; it has artifically segmented skills so that needed services, like health care, are increasingly difficult to supply economically; it has fostered the cynical view that unethical practices will prevail unless those entrenched in a profession are assured of high incomes; and it has caused a proliferation of official administrative bodies, most of them staffed by persons drawn from and devoted to furthering the interests of the licensed occupations themselves. [pp. 16-18]

Haberfield et al. (1978) noted a growing movement directed at regulatory reform. Though there was little agreement about what shape this reform should take, there did appear to be some agreement to question whether licensing agencies were achieving the purpose of protecting the public. A related question was whether there was undue restriction on the market-place without offsetting benefit to the public welfare.

Three ways of dealing with the questions of reform appear to be evident. First, there are those who argue that there is too much government in our lives. Regulatory agencies are seen to be outmoded, unneeded, and too costly and should be revamped or terminated. The sunset review laws, about which something will be said later in this chapter, are examples of an outgrowth of this argument. A second group basically approves of the idea of regulation but believes current regulation is insufficient. They perceive regulation to be either irrelevant or less stringent than is necessary to protect the needs of the public. They argue against regulation based on professional "self-policing." A third group focuses on the structural and procedural shortcomings of regulation which have resulted in unfair, preferential, prejudicial, and delayed treatment of public protection problems. Though there tends to be some agreement that licensing agencies have lost touch with the needs of the public (indeed, if they have ever been in touch), this group questions whether and to what extent they can be made accountable. Some argue that the bureaucratization of licensing has gone so far that licensing agencies respond more to their own needs for survival than to the special interests of the professionals they regulate or to the needs of the public. Others hold that regulation is inherently contradictory. By limiting the availability of service, the competition between care givers, consumer choices, and industry innovation, regulation reduces these quality-generating factors for the supposed purpose of achieving higher quality. This suggests that the essential problem regulators must solve, according to

Haberfield et al. (1978), "is to insure that the social costs of such regulation do not so outweigh its perceived benefits as to render its continuation burdensome and without merit" (p. A5).

Hopewell's (1980) criticism of regulation cuts somewhat more deeply by focusing on the system as participating in the production of self-defeating results. Very little guidance is available to licensing board members and few practical limits (other than the usually distracted state legislature) are available on their rule-making power. The breadth of the scope of the statutes and vagueness of the criteria to judge the adequacy of rules adopted permit vast latitude for developing and for justifying almost any action short of violating the Constitution. The lack of coordination of licensing agencies, their failure to attract media attention, and the absence of an office to provide ongoing supervision means that the power of licensing agencies is virtually unchecked. Board members thrust into this situation, mostly oriented by their experience to the needs of the profession being regulated, uneducated about theories of regulation or economics, and unprepared to serve as regulators, will tend to be uncritical about their pro-profession biases. It is inevitable in Hopewell's (1980) view that this system "is a prescription for generation of poor regulatory decisions" (p. 3). Breyer (1980), defending the system, noted that there are limits in the administrative procedures acts which require advance notice of decision, the right of parties affected by decision to a hearing, and the provision of publicly recorded reasons for decisions. Further, he pointed out that agencies must act in a way they can later justify in a court of law where reviews of agency decision making may very well be taken.

Regulatory Models

The forms of regulation are varied, but Breyer (1980) identified five theoretical types of regulatory programs that are concerned with the quality of service rather than with the control of prices or regulation of the quality of products.

1. *Allocation under a public interest standard* occurs when regulators allocate a limited number of licenses among competing applicants. The regulator's job is to determine which applicants best meet the public interest criteria. To make this judgment the regulator must develop criteria for judgment and a system to get the data needed to make a judgment. In this form of regulation the problem is to find objective standards in situations that often call for subjective judgments. In effect, some standards will give preference to one set of providers over another. Often the best judgments are those that subjectively review and weigh a variety of criteria, yet the basis for the judgment may remain unclear, the judgments from one time to the next inconsistent, and the judgments exposed to criticism of "politics."

2. *In historically based allocation regulation*, the criteria are based on past

experience. It circumvents the complexities of dealing with public interest criteria though there is a built-in obsolescence requiring an increasing need to make exceptions to remedy inequities, which in turn makes the system more complex.

3. *Standard setting* seeks to control adverse effects by identifying particular causal elements. Standards are written that maximize the limitation of adverse effects and minimize undesirable side effects. In actual practice this process is fraught with complications. The definition of both adverse effects and causal elements are subject to political debate, negotiation between the affected parties, and long delays due to foot-dragging and difficulties in clarifying what is to be regulated. An adversarial relationship between the standards setters and the regulated industry causes difficulty in obtaining accurate and complete information about the standards. Enforcement is a second problem of standard setting. Applicability of standards (so they can be enforced by staff) often competes with their relevance (the standards may be so simple they do not effectively make the standard operational). Standards may increase competition between providers, may restrict entry of new providers, and may favor some providers over others. Standards must also be able to survive judicial review.

4. *Individual screening* is the type of regulation typicaly applied to the selection of individual licensees to serve the public. A case-by-case approach, in effect, compares applicant qualifications to the criteria set by regulation. Precision of standards, expensive testing procedures, circumstances that lead to highly subjective judgments, conflicts of interest, gaining adequate information, determining the benefits and risks of provider procedures, differential application of criteria, and the requirements of judicial review all pose problems in implementing this approach to regulation.

5. *Disclosure regulation* helps consumers to make more informed choices. Regulators set standards about what should be disclosed, how and where the disclosures should take place, and how the standards will be enforced. The problems of information, enforcement, competition, and judicial review are also involved here. Disclosure regulation has the advantage of not restricting or interfering with provider flexibility or consumer choice. As a result, the problems of implementation are less difficult to solve, the standards are easier to write, and the results are more successful and efficient than when compared with alternative regulating efforts. Disclosure requires a consumer population that can understand the information and is free to choose on the basis of the information.

Theories of Regulation

Theories of regulation primarily focus on explaining regulatory agency behavior. Early theory emphasized structural factors, comparing the cohesion of the regulated group to the amorphousness of the public. This leads to a circumstance where little is done that is not acceptable to the regulated group. Stigler (1971) observed that "every industry or occupation that has enough political power to utilize the state will seek to control entry" (p. 5).

Bernstein (1955) proposed a life cycle model of regulatory agencies. First, there is a period characterized by organized pressure on the legislature for reform of an existing situation followed by the initial statutory mandate. The agency then struggles to gain stability and permanence by fighting for support for its budget and appropriate legal authority. In most cases, the only ongoing interest at this time in how it is faring will come from the regulated group. The initial reformist zeal and popular support (if any) declines precipitously following the legislative mandate. The agency then enters a period of debility and decline. To quote Cohen (1975), it becomes a captive of the regulated groups. "The agency is thus converted, over time, from functioning as a check on the regulated interest to that of an ally or even subsidiary of the nominal subject of regulation" (p. 123).

There appear to be differences between those agencies that result from regulated groups seeking regulation and those originating in the efforts of a third party. They generally differ in the extent to which members of the regulated group are part of the regulatory agency. Nonetheless, Cohen (1975) presents an analysis of the Peer Standards Review Organizations program to support his view that "the basic cues for regulatory agency behavior may be found in the initial legislative struggles" (p. 125).

Wilson (1980) argued for a politics of regulation. He believed legislators were vote maximizers who dealt with problems of scarcity and conflicting preferences by arbitrating amongst competing interests so that no "adversary party gets all it wants; each is optimally disgruntled" (p. 361). He looked to explain regulatory agency behavior by describing the motives of the types of employees who make up their staffs.

Careerists identify themselves with the agency, not expecting rewards or jobs from external constituencies. Their first concern is the maintenance of the agency. They avoid risk as their comfort, security, and prospects could be threatened by a crisis or scandal. Security is preferred to rapid growth, autonomy is desired rather than competition, and stability is valued more than change. They do not wish to be associated with negative occurrences, or criticized for doing "nothing," and their great fear is they may be ridiculed. They attempt to minimize the conditions leading to catastrophe or absurdity by extensive rule making. Properly referred to as "covering your flanks," Wilson (1980) identified the "tar-baby" effect: "regulations tend to multiply owning to the unanticipated consequences of any given regulation" (p. 377). Wilson hypothesized risk avoidance rather than imperialism or power acquisition to explain the proliferation of rule making by careerists.

When *politicians* are employees their motives are bound up in their future, or lack of it, in elective or appointive office outside the agency. Wilson's (1980) analysis separated the politicians for whom the appointment was a dead end from those for whom it was a launching pad. Those rewarded for past political favors may be older persons on their way down or younger persons going nowhere. They will tend to act like careerists but may cater more to the regulated industry. Unidentified with the agencies as the careerists are and having no serious political ambition or professional identification, they are most susceptible to such potential economic rewards as well-paying positions after retirement from public service or special favors while in public service. On the other hand, politicians who have a future in politics have found it politically useful to identify with the needs of consumers. Their actions tend to reflect a suspicion of institutions and a critical view of business and other providers.

Professionals are primarily motivated by the prospect of the esteem of other professionals. Whether they hope to stay with the agency or leave it, they do expect to remain in the ranks of the profession, thus their behavior will not stray very far from behavior approved by the profession and its definition of professional competence. Since professional norms are the primary reference for behavior, they may lead an agency to regulate either more or less aggressively than they otherwise might. Some professionals who identify with the agency more than the profession will act like careerists.

Though a given agency staff member may have more than one of these motives, Wilson (1980) expected to find politicians most heavily represented among the top executives, careerists most heavily represented at the middle-manager level, and professionals were most likely to be found at the operational level. In the agencies he studied he found coalitions of differently motivated participants with tension and change expressed in the competition among these staff members.

In reviewing the nature of change in regulatory environments, Wilson (1980) saw the prospects for change enhanced by the introduction of new technology or because of changes in the larger environment. The price of health care and the proliferation of licensed occupations have stimulated much new interest and questioning in the licensing of professionals, while new technology is largely responsible for the proliferation of licensed occupations. The cost of political access has lessened recently as political action groups are sustained by foundations, computerized direct-mail fund drives, media interest, and court cost reimbursements, allowing them to lobby in legislative halls and enter the courts to challenge agency decisions. More extensive judicial review of agency functioning has occurred as a result. In concluding, Wilson (1980) noted:

the largely unsupervised nature of most regulatory activity . . . the absence of good evidence that there is a clear statutory solution to the problems that beset these agencies . . . [and] that much of what appears to be the result of bureaucratic ineptitude, agency imperialism, or political meddling is the result of the sheer magnitude of many regulatory tasks. . . . A single-explanation theory of regulatory politics is about as helpful as a single explanation of politics generally, or of disease. [pp. 391-93]

Change

Change is an agony in regulatory systems where the prevailing motif is inertia; where innovation is swallowed up by systems enormously resistant to change; and where the energy of reformers is co-opted by structure, time, and innovation without change. Of the recommendations of the 1971 U.S. Department of Health, Education, and Welfare *Report on Licensure and Related Health Personnel Credentialing* (HSM 72-11), only one called for structural change in occupational licensing. Institutional licensure was suggested as an alternative to a proliferation of the complexity, fragmentation, and inadequacy of the state-by-state control of licensing personnel. There had been much experience with institutional licensing of facilities, so the report recommended the initiation of demonstration projects focused on personnel. The idea was to locate the responsibility for competency assessment in an institution, thereby providing a regulatory framework for the encouragement of team approaches to service and of integrating new kinds of personnel. Though there were some demonstration projects, the institutional licensure idea was torpedoed by the professions fearful of losing their separate identities (and their special status within the institutions) and of becoming subservient to nonprofessional administrators who would, under institutional licensing, have ultimate authority to make professional decisions.

The idea for sunset laws was recommended, also in 1971, by the New Jersey Professional and Occupational Study Commission. The state of Colorado passed the first sunset law in 1976 and by 1981 thirty-five states had them. Although the HEW report had been stimulated primarily by the proliferation of occupational licensing, sunset laws grew out of the concern for accountability in the administration of economic regulation and public service. Sunset laws change the way state governments have conducted their oversight and budgetary responsibilities. Instead of assuming that agencies will continue operating until a legislature decides to stop them, agencies, under sunset laws, automatically terminate unless a legislature agrees to continue them. Sunset laws are procedures that tip the scales, in the problem of proliferation and effectiveness of governmental activities, from inertia to change as Moore (1980) has said, since "It is always more likely that a legislature will fail to act rather than take a controversial step. Sunset shifts the burden of proof from those advocating termination to those advocating continuation" (p. 31).

The way sunset provisions generally work is that a timetable is set in advance for the review of particular state agencies. The agencies are designated for termination on designated dates (usually by statute). Only the legislature can act to reestablish the agency and then only for a specified period of time, at the end of which the agency is again reviewed. Gathering data for the review is left to a sunset commission. Tochen (1978) noted the criteria included in the Florida Regulatory Reform Act of 1976.

• Would the absence of regulation significantly harm or endanger the public health, safety, or welfare?

- Is there a reasonable relationship between the exercise of the state's police power and the protection of the public health, safety, or welfare?
- Is there another less restrictive method of regulation available which could adequately protect the public?
- Does the regulation have the effect of directly or indirectly increasing the costs of any goods or services involved, and if so, to what degree?
- Is the increase in cost more harmful to the public than the harm which could result from the absence of regulation?
- Are all facets of the regulatory process designed solely for the purpose of or have as their primary effect, the protection of the public? [p. 28]

Martin's (1980) study of sunset review in 1977-1978, shown in table 6.4, reveals an early pattern of heavy termination recommendations (46.6 percent) but in the states where action was taken, a disregard of these recommendations by the state legislatures was found. Only 17.5 percent of the recommendations were followed. Twice as many boards were modified as were recommended to be modified while eighteen times as many boards were continued without modification than were recommended. In the states where action was delayed, the proportion of terminations recommended was less than half, while modification recommendations doubled, and continuance recommendations tripled. Martin (1980) concluded, "for those who saw in sunset legislation the opportunity to break the monopoly hold of professional occupations by terminating large numbers of occupational licensing boards, the evidence thus far has not been encouraging" (p. 148).

Martin (1980) theorized that a combination of extensive lobbying by regulated groups and the difficulty in estimating indirect costs of licensing (which leads the legislature to ignore these costs) combine to explain the failure of sunset legislation to have much of an effect on occupational licensing. Since future sunset reviews will consider such prestigious occupations as law, medicine, dentistry, architecture, accounting, and optometry, all of which have large indirect components to the cost of regulation, he did not expect this conclusion to change much. He believed the most important modification that will be made will be to include public representatives on licensing boards.

The Common Cause study (Stephens, 1982) of sunset is more positive in seeing improvements in governmental performance. Approximately 60 percent of the states responding reported that recommendations of sunset commissions are accepted by state legislators 76 to 100 percent of the time. Of almost 1,500 agencies reviewed between 1976 and 1981, 18 percent were terminated, 38 percent were modified, and 44 percent were recreated without change. The major reason, according to the report, that recommendations were not followed was pressure from professional associations. A 1980 workshop (Roederer and Palmer, 1981), which intensively studied six health licensing boards (chiropractors, dentists, physicians, nurses, psy-

**TABLE 6.4 Disposition of Occupational Licensing Boards under
Select Sunset Legislation, 1977-1978 (Fifteen States)**

	Recommended	Action taken	
Nine States where disposition occurred			
Termination	37 (68.5%)	21 (17.5%)	
Action as a percentage of recommendation			(56.8%)
Modification	13 (24.1%)	25 (20.8%)	
Action as a percentage of recommendation			(192.3%)
Continuance	4 (7.4%)	74 (61.7%)	
Action as a percentage of recommendation			(1,850.0%)
	54 (100%)	120 (100.0%)	
Six States where disposition was delayed			
Termination	17 (27.4%)		
Modification	32 (51.6%)		
Continuance	13 (21.0%)		
	62 (100.0%)		
Total Recommendations			
Termination	54 (46.6%)		
Modification	45 (38.7%)		
Continuance	17 (14.7%)		
	116 (100.0%)		

Source: Donald L. Martin, "Will the Sun Set on Occupational Licensing?" in S. Rottenberg, ed., *Occupational Licensure and Regulation* (Washington, D.C.: American Enterprise Institute, 1980), p. 147.

chologists, veterinarians) in six states, was also more positive indicating that "very few agencies or boards were eliminated. Instead, sunset reviews produced changes in management and operational practices" (p. 11).

Tochen (1978) reported another factor involved in the effectiveness of sunset review. The cost of the review process itself is high. He reported that in Colorado the state auditor was required to prepare a performance audit prior to agency termination dates. For thirteen agencies in 1977, the cost per agency for this one aspect of the review process averaged over $10,000. This drain on state fiscal resources can be extensive, making continued financing problematic. Moore (1980) mentioned the heavy workload that sunset review stimulated and the fact that it was so heavily influenced by political considerations where conflicting constituencies influence the process. He noted in this regard that legislators were reluctant to take the automatic termination step because it was a step they saw as extreme. It is a case of enthusiasm for the idea in general but not in the specific. The major virtue of sunset review was seen as having taken occupational licensing boards out of the hidden corridors of state government and brought back into the limelight. Having to periodically justify the mission in public, even though agency members and executives know that their agency is protected by the regulated group's lobbying efforts, opens their eyes and may curb the more obvious abuses and the most irrelevant agencies.

Gordon (1980) saw the improvement of regulation as coming from greater clarity and specificity. He suggested regulators ask these questions:

1. What *exactly* is to be regulated?
2. How will success be measured?
3. What is required to bring all parties involved to a concensus concerning:
   a. The need for regulation
   b. The regulatory mode or approach most appropriate to secure the ends desired?
4. How will activities be monitored to ensure that regulatory ends are achieved?
   a. Are budgetary provisions adequate to do the job?
   b. Even with an adequate budget, are there trained persons available to execute monitoring programs?
5. What system will be instituted for testing and evaluating alternative intervention schemes?
6. What approach will be used to identify and correct problems that emerge once the regulatory program takes effect?
7. Can all those involved or with a stake in the regulatory proposal be identified? Can their objectives and concerns also be identified?
   a. Regulatory entities?
   b. Executive and legislative branch political overseers?
   c. Executives and administratives with related responsibilities in public or private agencies?
   d. Regulated organizations and associations?
   e. Community and public interest groups including;
      1. Those with trustee or fiduciary oversight?
      2. Consumers including their own health resource providers— (employers, insurance companies, etc.)? [pp. 354-55]

The Roederer and Palmer (1981) workshop concluded on the note of accountability. They asked that the following data be made available by licensing boards generally so as to study the impact of licensing boards, their regulations, and the sunset review process.

- number of health professionals per 1,000 (and ultimately the increase or decrease per capita of professionals per 1,000); location of practitioners; case loads
- percentage of applicants who pass licensing exams
- percentage of foreign applicants who apply for and are granted licensure
- percentage of out-of-state applicants who apply for and are granted licensure
- number of consumer complaints
- percentage of consumer complaints which result in investigations and disciplinary actions
- time required to resolve disciplinary actions
- number of disciplinary cases which result in revocations vs. other penalties
- number of professionals involved in continuing education
- impact of continuing education on service quality
- amount of license fees
- revenue generated by fees vs. administrative costs of licensing [p. 13]

Their suggestions stand as mute testimony of the inadequate knowledge about an enterprise that affects the American society so profoundly. That this information is not generally available and that, with one minor exception, the information requested relates to the process of regulating, not its outcome, argues against the position that licensing boards protect the public. The following chapters examine the record of licensing boards relative to public protection and suggest some of the dimensions that must be considered if greater public protection is to become an eventuality.

7

DEFINING COMPETENCE

Questions about competency and quality quickly raise some very complicated issues. Pottinger (1979c) indicated the can of definitional worms one can get into when serious concern is raised about the failure of traditional credentials to relate to quality performance of service to the public.

Assuming for the moment that professionals are genuinely interested in protecting the public through licensure, the question of what constitutes protection must be clearly addressed. Let us assume we can come to some decision about this. Once consensus is reached about what constitutes protection, it becomes an empirical matter to determine how this is best achieved. One critical aspect of determining what works best will be the proper identification of the knowledge, skills, abilities, and other characteristics that define necessary minimal levels of competence. After these competencies have been identified they must be empirically linked to outcomes; and finally, a means of measuring these qualities reliably, validly, and meaningfully is required. [p. 26]

Menne (1981) argued against competency-based assessment and discussed four of these difficulties for the profession of psychology: defining a psychologist's behavior in terms of task statements; the endless number of such tasks for the entire profession; the impossibility of defining a minimal level of competence for each task; and the small likelihood that any psychologist would perform at criterion level or above for all tasks. Such difficulties, the very way the problem of competence is defined, and past disinterest in assessing competence explain the past avoidance of Pottinger's (1979c) questions.

Licensure examinations ordinarily depend on tests of knowledge recall based on material learned in university classrooms. These tests have not been found to be related to acceptable performance in a profession. It would require much energy from professional groups and the public to address and gain consensus on defining the purpose of protection (Protect whom?

Against what? For minimal competency or high quality? For how long?) and to clarify competency measures in ways meaningful to public protection. Further, the California Board of Medical Quality Assurance proposal (1982) indicated the necessity that standards of competence require agreement on these issues:

What does the practice consist of; what tasks, activities or modalities are involved; what cognitive and affective knowledge and skills are critical to being able to do these things; what are the consequences of lack of these knowledges and skills; are those consequences sufficiently hazardous to make the absence of competence critical; what educational or training experiences are essential to attaining competence, and are these viable alternatives; can competence be measured, and if so how; who is competent to make valuations of the competence of practitioners; how can outcomes of treatment be evaluated . . . ? [pp. 23-24]

The problems with present systems of credentialing suggest that neither public protection nor competency have been of primary concern, as we have indicated previously. But in response to criticism of the professions and licensing arrangements, court cases (*Griggs* v. *Duke Power Company*, 1971), and equal opportunity federal guidelines, there has been a renewed interest in understanding the nature of competence. In this chapter the problems involved in the present forms of credentialing competence will be addressed, and then some of the changing ideas about competence over time will be described.

LIMITED AND INVALID CREDENTIALS

Test results are involved directly in providing the data necessary for educational diplomas and degrees. The major problem posed by traditional paper and pencil tests of knowledge is that they tap only a very small part of the richness of human behavior. Such tests predominate in the credentials industry. McGuire (1969) posed the problem as it refered to the education of physicians.

Current systems of student examination, grading and promotion, and those of physician licensure and certification not only fail to provide evidence regarding achievement with respect to many of the most important goals of medical education, but actually jeopardize their attainment by exacerbating tendencies toward fragmentation of learning, by focusing attention on esoteric or trivial detail, and by intensifying unhealthy competition among students for grades and among specialities for trainees' time and attention. . . . Such measurement would be defensible if it could be shown that these techniques yield accurate, dependable results which are highly correlated with . . . physicians' performance. Unfortunately such is not the case. Studies at all educational levels monotonously reveal, first, that the examination techniques characteristic of medical educators yield such unreliable individual scores that little confidence can be placed in them and second, that even when great care is taken to minimize common sources of error, performance on typical tests at either undergraduate or specialty board levels bears little relation to effective practice. [p. 593]

Pottinger (1977) used an analogy to make the same point—measuring how fast someone can drink by requiring them to use a straw. Both the "paper and pencil test and the straw . . . limit the phenomenon being measured in a reliable way" (p. 10).

One dimension of richness in human behavior is the variety of ways people are able to solve identical problems. In this way people with competent skills in one area (for example, logical analysis) are sometimes able to compensate for deficiencies in other areas (for example, reading speed). A variety of different levels of performance could add up to an adequate overall performance level. In the licensing examination situation, arbitrary norms are usually set to determine the passing grade. Even in examinations that test multiple areas of knowledge, the arbitrariness of bureaucratic judgment often creates ridiculous circumstances. Augustine (1979) cited the case of the podiatrist who failed an examination requiring both a seventy-five average and a score no less than 60 on a subpart. Though the podiatrist maintained a 75 average for all the subparts, he received a fifty-eight in one part and failed the exam. In response to suggestions that there ought to be a "gray area" (for example, fifty-five to sixty) where other factors could be used to pass an application, Augustine raised the question of the "bottom line." What do you do then with the person who scores a 54.4? And so on. And so on. But this is the kind of discussion that is inevitable given the narrow content focus for measurement and the resulting arbitrary standards that support such a focus.

The traditional examination may very well be reliable, that is, measure whatever phenomenon it examines with consistency. But just because a test reliably measures the knowledge that is the basis for practice does not mean that the test is reporting valid information, that is, information relevant to acceptable performance. Klemp (1979) reported:

The way competence is ascribed to a person and the way it is measured, however, are often two different things. Somewhere along the line psychologists defined certain knowledge, skills and personality traits and developed measures for them. They found that these measures often corresponded with judgments of competency and decided, therefore, that the measures and the competency were the same thing. Granted, it appears that test scores, college grades, and career performance inventories do predict entrance into a given occupation. Nevertheless, once a person enters that occupation none of those measures will reliably predict that person's performance. [p. 41]

Nor is there comfort that traditional measures predict entrance into an occupation. This is more the consequence of the political use of the credentialing system to bar entry to occupations than the adequacy of the prediction formula. The predictability is so good with regard to entry because the measures both express and maintain the social class and racial composition of members of occupations. To increase performance predictability the measures would have to sample behavior actually related to practice, a change that might very well alter the social class and racial composition of the members of an occupation. The foot-dragging on making measurement of competency relevant to practice is undoubtedly related to the threat of displacement.

In the health and human services areas, particularly, the problem of relevance has been exacerbated by the ambiguity of the goals. There is little agreement about defining what "health" is, for example. Without a clear picture of the objective to be achieved it is not really possible to determine the degree of competency of a practitioner's performance, since it is not known what it is the practitioner should be accomplishing. Operational definitions develop that may vary from one situation to another according to the values of the definer or according to what can be most easily measured or both. Given the narrow way definitions of "competence" have been put into operation in the professions (for example, most tests of knowledge), it seems clear that there will be persons who presently meet the criteria whose practice is incompetent when judged by performance standards. There also will be those who presently do not meet the criteria but whose practice would be considered competent according to performance standards. Carl Rogers (1973) was most sensitive to the existence of the latter.

I think of the "hot-line" workers I have been privileged to know in recent years. They handle, over the phone, bad drug trips, incipient suicides, tangled love affairs, family discord, all kinds of personal problems. Most of these workers are college students or just beyond this level, with minimal intensive "on-the-job" training. And I know that in many of these crisis situations they use a skill and judgment that would make a professional turn green with envy. They are completely "unqualified," if we use conventional standards. But they *are*, by and large, both dedicated and *competent*. [p. 382]

As a result, a situation presently exists whereby professions have used entrance criteria that ensure a continued flow of qualified but not necessarily competent persons into the professions. It is all very well to say that this circumstance should be changed, but changing credentialing criteria for continued or new membership means that many persons accustomed to being rewarded with money, status, and security for certain behaviors, attitudes, and knowledge will no longer be so rewarded. Instead, others would take their places. Such a "changing of the guard" is never accomplished easily and is rarely accomplished without some pain, resistance, hostility, and even bloodshed in extreme cases. After all, credentialing does turn out to be a "bread and butter" issue where the "ins" get theirs and the "outs" do not. Therefore, a major problem in this area is that defining credentialing criteria is not just an academic exercise. It has real-life implication and drama affecting millions of people and scores of large and economically and politically powerful institutions. It cuts into our more deeply set expectations about success and failure in life.

CHANGING NOTIONS ABOUT COMPETENCY

Modern life began to become exceedingly complicated because of industrialization, centralization, and mass production toward the close of the nineteenth century. In earlier and simpler times, the artisan and the professional were known personally to consumers by the fruits of their labors over time within the context of a coherent community. Thus, performance was ordinarily monitored by people who knew the professional personally. They frequently communicated informally with other persons in their community, informing them about the quality of performance. Credentialing was highly personal and concretely related to the necessary social encounters of the time. A family name had meaning in this system and served as a symbol for reliability and integrity. But with the increased congregating of persons in large numbers in anonymous cities, this personal credentialing system was no longer adequate for an increasing number of competency judgments that had to be made not only by consumers but by the increasingly large institutions that ordered societal life. Though education as an institution had long provided a credential in the academic degree, it did not take on the significance it now has until the beginning of the twentieth century. (See discussion in chapter 4 about this period.) It is part of America's mythology to value the man "who pulled himself up by his own bootstraps," but the pride of individual accomplishment through hard work and sterling performance began to give way at this time to a recognition of the importance of education. How much a person knew began to be taken for an indication of a person's ability to perform well, and at still another level of abstraction diplomas and degrees became a substitute for knowledge. Beginning during the first world war, the Army Alpha spurred the testing movement by providing a paper and pencil "intelligence" test. Such credentials eventually had the effect of replacing accomplishment with an achievement test score, ability with an intelligence quotient, and motivation with an interest inventory. As a consequence the subjective evaluation of personal knowledge was replaced by an "objective" credential—a widely understood code for competence, much as the American Express card is for consumption.

Like some social movements, these changes were associated with egalitarian sentiments. As personal as prior definitions of competency were, they were also overlaid with a social class bias that favored a landed, monied class and perpetuated an untitled aristocracy, particularly in the settled regions of the United States. The frontier, by necessity, had been the location for a more egalitarian- and performance-oriented definition of competence. With the decline of the frontier and the impact of industrialization, changes began to occur in the concepts of competence and the means of assessing it. According to Pottinger (1980a), at the beginning of the twentieth century intelligence became associated with merit and testing with the allocation of opportunity.

Intelligence testing exploded into popular acceptability and use not because of its scientific merits, but because it could be seized on as part of a fair and just system of social contracts. The assumption was that intelligence was a fairer criterion for social status than aristocracy, and that an intelligence test was an appropriate measure of this criterion. [p. 16]

We need not detail here all the products of the intelligence-testing explosion, but it has dominated our conceptions of competence for the last eighty years. Intelligence testing predicted and determined success in school and college, and these institutions became the gateway to a new system of cultural stratification that has controlled entry into life opportunity. In asking the questions about what intelligence tests predict, McClelland's (1973) answer was:

Certainly they are valid for predicting who will get ahead in a number of prestige jobs where credentials are important. So is white skin: it too is a valid predictor of job success in prestige jobs. But no one would argue that white skin per se is an ability factor. Lots of the celebrated correlations between so-called intelligence test scores and success can lay no greater claim to representing an ability factor. [p. 6]

The credentialing system based on measured intelligence has had the effect of pushing along toward high achievement particular elements of the population and restraining others. According to McClelland (1973):

Belonging to the power elite (high socioeconomic status) not only helps a young man go to college and get jobs through contacts his family has, it also gives him easy access as a child to the credentials that permit him to get into certain occupations. Nowadays, those credentials include the words and word-game skills used in scholastic aptitude tests. In the Middle Ages they required knowledge of Latin for the learned professions of law, medicine, and theology. [p. 6]

Although individuals with the "right" intelligence test scores and educational credentials have prestigious opportunities open up to them, others without these brilliant credentials might also do well in life performance. Some persons, then, especially those from families with higher social class standing and with white skin, have been able to surmount the barriers placed in their way. In this regard, McClelland (1973) examined during the decade of the 1960s the accomplishments of two groups of elite (Wesleyan) university undergraduates he had in class in the 1940s—straight A students and C— students. He raised the question of the consequences of restrictiveness based on credentials.

To my great surprise, I could not distinguish the two lists of men 15-18 years later. There were lawyers, doctors, research scientists, and college and high school teachers in both groups. The only difference I noted was that those with better grades got into better law or medical schools, but even with this supposed advantage they did not have notably more successful careers as compared with the poorer students who had to be satisfied with "second-rate" law and medical schools at the outset. Doubtless the C— students could not get into even second rate law and medical schools under the stricter admissions testing standards of today. Is that an advantage for society? [p. 2]

The essential rightness of a classification system based on measured intelligence was accepted without much question for a period of sixty years. Measured intelligence defined our conceptions of competence and ordered our institutions. But beginning with the civil rights struggles of the 1960s, the flaw inherent in the measured intelligence credential became obvious— "not everyone of potentially equal merit had an equal opportunity to develop intellectually" (Pottinger, 1980a, p. 16). Collins (1979) believed this reevaluation emanated from an inflationary devaluation of educational credentials, high school graduation becoming near-universal and college graduation commonplace. An initial result was a loss of appeal of these goals as they no longer guaranteed a respectable job after high school or an elite one after college. This factor, together with pressure from blacks and Spanish-language ethnic groups for entry into the credentialing system, produced a confidence crisis. Questions were raised loudly for the first time about the restrictions on opportunity and lack of relevance of the measured intelligence-based credentialing system. Attempts to tinker with the system with collegiate open admissions policies and curricular reforms failed to substantially change the system. Following the relevance crisis of the 1960s, college students are more cynical than ever in their acceptance of credentialism. They recognize that the credentialing system continues to be the primary pathway to a decent job. There are still doubts raised: employers receive pressure from the courts for selection tests to be job related; there are demands for accountability from the public; and legislators block licensing new occupations where there is not evident public need. These interventions, however, still only tinker with the system relying as they do on traditional credentials. Any system of reform must provide alternative occupational pathways that do what the present, measured intelligence-based system does—integrate with the economic system by tying the pathway to the job structure and linking education and vocation.

THE MEASUREMENT OF COMPETENCY

The neglect of competency assessment by the professions has not just been for the lack of theory and research but rather a lack of resources and will. Erdmann (1976) discussed specialty certification examinations for physicians:

It seems within the power of the Boards to define board certified status as representing only advanced knowledge in a given specialty. On the other hand, it could specifically be intended to have implications for the quality of care one is likely to receive from physicians achieving the designation. Obviously, the measurement problems are at almost opposite extremes of the continuum of feasibility. The knowledge evaluation is a relatively easy task. The prediction of quality of care is another matter altogether and pushes the state of the art of measurement at the current time beyond its capacity to respond in a definitive fashion. . . . A reasonable question is "why is this problematic?" Given ideal circumstances and endless resources, it of course is not. Realistically, however, resources are limited and conditions far from ideal. The danger then becomes one of mounting a massive validation effort only to discover that a good part of it is very difficult if not impossible, with the result that the evidence which tends to be developed is that which is easiest to obtain and least expensive. [pp. 19-20]

We, however, often have the energy, time, and money for goals we consider important. As we previously indicated, what we measure and do not measure is a demonstration of particular values and an instrument of social policy. Heaton (1977) made this point in writing about the relationship of measurement to productivity of service organizations.

Measurement is purposeful, not neutral; shaped by social structure, not independent; distorted by intellectual conventions, not unbiased. . . . Things that are not measured are not controlled. By not measuring the productivity of organizations in serving people, we have relinquished control over organizations. [p. 37]

Anne Paxton (1982) reviewed the procedures involved in determining the competency of airplane pilots. She concluded:

Where performance is important to us, we naturally expect rigorous guarantees of competence, we impose sanctions such as decertification on those who fail to meet the standards, and we don't put a lot of faith in self-regulation. Compare the public's tolerance toward the medical profession which admits that up to 10 percent of its members are drug addicts or alcoholics. . . . It is possible that we really don't care whether physicians are competent—or could it be that we are so unsure of what constitutes competence in medicine that we couldn't evaluate it if we wanted to? And if so, hadn't we better wonder whether there's a reason for licensing physicians—or any other profession—at all? [p. 11]

La Duca (1980) engaged in investigations of competency assessment. His work led him to conclude that the problem is not just of methodology but of paradigm. The trait model of problem-solving on which some researchers have relied in their work ignores the crucial element that our reality is situation specific.

Human behavior in professional occupations occurs in a "real world" of persons, places, and things. Unfortunately, it has become traditional to define professional competence as behavior isolated from these circumstances, reflecting a surrender to the seductiveness of behavioral inventories. Ultimately, the price is limited utility. [p. 254]

Instead, he offered the idea that "professional competence exists as collective manifestations of situational responses" (p. 255). The path for research led away from intrapsychic constructs which were collectively thought to represent competence to a study of the environment of practice—the relationships between the perceiving professional and the client, the problem, and the setting. The professional actively interprets input from situational patterns. The result is a purposive perception of meaning and behaviors in the situation. He concluded:

This is not to say that the situation determines behaviors. Rather, the relationship seems to be closer to one where the encountered circumstances establish the parameters for behaviors. . . . The "heart" of behavior, especially that which constitutes professional competence is to be found neither totally in the person nor totally in the situation. It is, instead, in the *relationship* between the two. [p. 285]

Investigations using his Professional Performance Situations Model (PPSM) will be described later in this chapter.

Competency measurement is ultimately tied to evaluation of the fitness of professionals to perform a service at an agreed upon level or standard. Competency itself is a construct, never seen directly, but rather observed in the behavior or the performance of the professional. Judgments are made about the knowledge, skill, and wisdom of a professional on the basis of particular acts in specific circumstances. Shimberg (1983) distinguished between competence and performance: competence had a future connotation while performance was viewed after the fact, though performance could be used as a competency predictor.

Boyatzis (1982) tied performance to competency:

Effective performance in a job can be defined as demonstrating a system and sequence of behaviors that produce the specific results required by the job while maintaining or being consistent with policies, procedures, and conditions of the organizational environment. The individual's competencies, the demands of the job, and the organizational environment must intersect. . . . [p. 223]

McGaghie (1980) referred to the content boundaries of competency as necessary to understand its meaning for a particular profession. "Content is the 'stuff' of professional practice, the knowledge and insight, skills and savvy, sentiments and dispositions that form the substance of professional work" (p. 295). Referring, then, to a person as competent inevitably means some reference to a circumscribed content domain but not content in its traditionally narrow sense. McGaghie urged "evaluators to look beyond inventories or discrete bits of knowledge and skill, and beyond personal traits . . . to include features of the social environment in domain descriptions to more fully capture professional practice" (p. 296).

Measurement is, essentially, systematic observation. Shimberg (1983) pointed out that competency assessment for licensure and certification began with direct observation of task performance on predetermined evaluation standards. Cost, time, insufficiency of task diversity, lack of equivalence in situations, and subjectivity of judges all have made the adequacy of direct observation somewhat problematic. He pointed out that standardized objective examinations broadened the content to be measured and made the assessment of different content areas equivalent with one another. Judgments about the content to be included, of course, remained subjective and it led to the use of job analyses to decide about content inclusion and emphasis. The state of the art has not taken standardized objective examinations much beyond assessing knowledge and understanding, though Shimberg discussed some interesting experimentation with problem solving and simulation, using computers rather than paper-and-pencil technology, and using a standardized task performance with videotape to provide data for evaluation.

The evaluation judgment that ultimately must be made can be such that those being evaluated are compared to each other (norm referenced) or compared to some standard of accomplishment (criterion referenced). Though licensing and certification examinations often have used norm referencing, the implication that the purpose of licensing is to bar entry to the incompetent argues for the use of criterion referencing. Norm referencing is seen to be more appropriate for employment selection where there would be competition among candidates for a limited number of positions. Criterion referencing requires a judgment of level or standard, which can be based on task and performance studies of the competencies needed by the practicing professional.

Two particular measurement problems are the assurance of *reliability* and *validity*. Reliability refers to the consistency of measures over time in yielding similar scores. Variations in scores can be introduced by the situation, the task or behavior being observed, the instrument, the scoring device, and the person utilizing the scoring method. A great deal of sophistication about reliability has resulted from work with objective, knowledge-oriented measures which may not be easily transferred to situational specific measurement. If the relationship between the perceiver and the situation is critical to this new approach to assessing professional competence and if these relationships are unique, this dimension poses serious problems for traditional views of reliability.

Measures might have excellent reliability but poor validity. Without validity in measures, evaluation is at best worthless and at worst irresponsible. The fact that a measure is not supported by evidence as to its utility (poor validity) has not always prohibited its use in assessment situations. Sometimes it seems on the face of it or to experts to represent what it is supposed to measure (*face validity*) and is, therefore, used without appraising its utility. When experts consider examination content important in preparation for a profession rather than performance of a service, this refers to the *content validity* of a measure. When a measure is highly related to some outcome of practice, this is called *criterion validity*. When a measure is compared with another measure known to distinguish low from high scoring professionals, this is called *concurrent validity*. When a measure predicts future high and low scorers on a performance measure, this is called *predictive validity*.

An American Psychological Association committee (1980) pointed out that criterion, content, and construct validity were not inseparable aspects nor discrete types of validity but rather differences in strategy in understanding the validity of measures.

Messick (1980) argued for the use of *construct validity*. Reliance on content and criterion validity is not enough; "the meaning of the measure must also be comprehended in order to appraise potential social consequences sensibly" (p. 1013). He defined construct validity as "a process of marshalling evidence to support the inference that an observed response consistency in test performance has a particular meaning, primarily by appraising the extent to which empirical relationships with other measures, or lack thereof, are consistent with that meaning" (p. 1015).

Kane's (1982) analysis of the issues relative to the validity of licensure exams is most pertinent. Differentiating between attempting to predict future professional performance and providing evidence on competence in specific critical abilities, he argued in favor of the latter. Though he did not use the same standards in evaluating the two approaches, his examination of the problems of achieving criterion or predictive validity and of the means to achieve content validity is useful. The essential problem with predictive validity is the difficulty of obtaining an adequate criterion. Suitable criterion selection is complicated by how to decide in the first place which criteria should be nominated as important to practice. Experts may be biased; studies of how professionals spend their time do not discriminate among activities in terms of their importance; and the critical-incident technique (which does emphasize perceived importance) does not provide a clear definition of professional competence. Assuming criteria could be developed, other problems exist. Client outcomes were rejected by Kane as inappropriate to compare with the criterion as these were contaminated by client characteristics which cannot be influenced by the practitioners; they introduced systematic error since the best practitioners may get the hardest cases; and they were inevitably based on small sample sizes which do not permit sufficient reliability. Similarly, process measures of criterion competency were rejected. Though ratings may be standardized, clients cannot be. Further,

professional practice involves a large number of activities in a wide variety of situations. The problems in developing a criterion are most serious for areas of practice involving a high degree of professional judgment, since a candidate's performance is likely to vary from one client to another, and expert raters may disagree on what the best action is in a particular situation. [p. 913]

Simulation examinations offer some possibilities but these too were rejected for their artificiality and lack of demonstrated relevance to professional performance. He did suggest that "ratings of performance are easiest to develop when the desired performance is simple and can be specified in detail" (p. 913). Finally, he noted the situational nature of competence requiring a large number of validity studies and the impossibility of developing an appropriate study as these would require performance evidence for failed candidates.

Arguing in favor of a content validity approach, Kane (1982) believed it more likely to gain evidence that would indirectly relate critical abilities to client outcomes. The ability would be examined in a large number of clinical trial situations to determine its relevance for professional practice. This approach would make possible the inclusion of these elusive abilities required in uncommon situations that would pose harm to the public if they were missed. Such an approach also had the advantage of being consistent with Equal Employment Opportunity Commission employment selection procedures. Kane's analysis can be interpreted as an argument against the possibility of measuring the overall competence of professionals and in favor of particular procedures as is suggested in chapter 9 if one takes the view that licensure exams should predict future professional performance. Kane rejected this purpose as setting up an unattainable standard but he did not provide evidence that examinations that evaluate critical abilities will correct the abuses noted in licensure examinations that have traditionally relied on content validity.

Since the topic of measurement is within the realm of psychology, it may be interesting to describe that profession's efforts to deal with the complexities of the validity problem. According to Schenkel (1980), the Examination Policy Committee of the American Association of State Psychology Boards had been struggling with a decision about whether to follow a content- or criterion-related validity model. At that time it appeared likely that the committee would choose the content-validity approach on the basis that "Psychologists work in diverse circumstances and the standards for the delivery of services vary widely" (p. 7). They did indicate that a good job analysis was necessary for adequate content validity. But even here there were members of the conference who argued against job analysis on the basis that as a method it has not developed sufficiently to permit an accurate description of the diversity of tasks psychologists perform. They feared reducing the field of psychology "to a number of simplified tasks which could be accomplished by anyone with sufficient in-service or on-the-job training and what would be lost is the identity and coherence of the profession of psychology" (p. 9). This group of psychologists would emphasize a generic knowledge base and the decisions psychologists make using this knowledge.

A job analysis usually describes the tasks or the behaviors involved in the performance of an occupation or profession (APA, 1980). Observation, interviews, TV taping, and reviewing performance standards and statements of objectives are some of the methods used. The approach may begin with identification of tasks performed in particular job classifications resulting in a behavioral description of each job classification. In another approach, attention is paid to job outputs. Following this, the knowledge and skill necessary to yield that product is described. Job definitions should then include the knowledge and skills necessary to perform the job, the tasks associated with that performance, and the situational context in which the performance takes place.

ATTEMPTS TO MEASURE COMPETENCY

The assessment center method of estimating job potential has its historical roots in the selection of personnel for Office of Strategic Services operations in World War II. Bray et al. (1974) described research using this method done for the American Telephone and Telegraph Company beginning in 1956. This research attempted to measure management potential of already recruited candidates for management positions. Table 7.1 delineates the twenty-five attributes studied (noting the correlations with later management program evaluations), the seven general characteristics that emerged from a factor analysis of the attributes data, and an indication of the assessment techniques primarily associated with each category of characteristics.

Later, Bray (1982) noted some flaws. The study did not examine such motives as money, status, or power that would impact on advancement. Also, the managers in the study did not include women or members of minority groups. The particular relevance of the study may be limited though the study is important as it indicated the utility of the assessment center method.

TABLE 7.1 Attributes of Management Potential and the Means by Which They Are Measured in an Assessment Center, Ranked according to Correlations with Management Progress Evaluations (N = 123)

Attributes	Factored Characteristics	Measured Primarily By
Oral communications skills (.33)*	Administrative skills	In-baskets
Human relations skills (.32)*	Interpersonal skills	Group exercises
Need for advancement (.31)*	Intellectual ability	Paper and pencil ability tests
Resistance to stress (.31)*	Stability of performance	Simulation exercises
Tolerance of uncertainty (.30)*	Work motivation	Projective tests, interviews, and simulation exercises
Organizing and Planning (.28)*		
Energy (.28)*	Career orientation	Projective tests and interviews
Creativity (.25)*	Dependency on others	Projective test
Range of interests (.23)*		
Behavior flexibility (.21)†		
Inner work standards (.21)†		
Need for security (−.20)†		
Scholastic aptitude (.19)†		
Ability to delay gratification (−.19)†		
Decision making (.18)†		
Primacy of work (.18)†		
Goal flexibility (−.18)†		
Perception of threshold Social Cues (.17)		
Need for approval of peers (−.17)		
Personal impact (.15)		
Need for approval of superiors (−.14)		
Social objectivity (.13)		
Realism of expectations (.08)		
Self-objectivity (.04)		
Bell System value orientation (−.02)		

Source: Douglas W. Bray, Richard J. Campbell, and Donald L. Grant, *Formative Years in Business: A Long-Term AT&T Study of Managerial Lives* (New York: Wiley. 1974), pp. 77-80.

*p<.01
†p<.05.

Klemp (1979) defined competency to include five generic characteristics of the person that are "causally related to effective behavior referenced to external performance criteria" (p. 42). Generic characteristics are manifested in various ways, in different situations, and with differing results. Included are: *knowledge* (organized information in a particular content area), *skill* (demonstration of related behaviors), *trait* (disposition to respond to an equivalent set of stimuli), *self-schema* (individual self-image and the self-evaluation of the image), and *motive* (ongoing concern for goals that drive, select, and direct individual behavior). These characteristics are integrated and interdependent in a holistic way so that one factor cannot be substituted for the whole. Finally, effectiveness is "defined by its relation to external performance criteria. This means, in part, that it is not sufficient that the individual be pleased with his or her own behavior —others also must deem it to be effective" (Klemp, 1979, p. 42). Klemp's definition of competence is oriented to the characteristics of the situation. Characteristics of the person in this case are not related in a simple way to characteristics of the situation, but are more broadly related to life and work outcomes.

Some definitions of competency assessment are so narrow that they set up self-imposed difficulties in measurement. Menne (1981), who argued against competency-based assessment for psychologists, defined it in the following way:

Competency based assessment measures the specific skills, behaviors, and information which are directly related to specific functions that will be performed by professional psychologists that demonstrate the ability of the professional psychologist to perform to criterion and function at a specified level. [p. 24]

Menne's task-based job analysis did not make reference to outcomes. A broader approach was described by Pottinger (1979c) who cited the example of United States Information Agency (USIA) officers whose job function required that they possess a high degree of communication skill. It was found that those USIA officers who were judged to be superior could communicate well because they had the ability to empathize with others and a strong positive disposition toward people.

McClelland and Boyatzis (1980) excluded from consideration in competency assessment those skills they call "threshold" skills. These are minimum skills required for a job, such as the ability to read and write, which do distinguish superior from average performers. These are considered skills but not competencies. Pottinger's (1979c) definition of competency has three parts: the interpersonal includes empathy, diagnostic listening, and faith in the ability of people to change; motivational attributes include the willingness to learn and the willingness to adapt to occupational requirements; and cognitive process abilities include seeing thematic consistencies in diverse information, organizing and communicating the different themes, conceptualizing the various sides of a controversial issue, and learning from experience.

Referring to the practice of medicine, McGuire (1963) hypothesized a six-level taxonomy of intellectual process which has an ascending order of competency. Level 1 included the recall of isolated information and the recognition of meaning or implication of performance. Level 2 involved the selection of generalizations to explain specific phenomena. Level 3 entailed making simple interpretations of data or applying principle to a familiar situation. Level 4 concerned the analysis of data or application of a unique combination of principles to a novel situation. Level 5 involved the evaluation of a total situation. Finally, level 6 required the analysis of a variety of elements of knowledge and application to a novel problem situation in its entirety.

The characteristics of the performance situation include working climates; job demands; the values, politics, and purposes involved in the situation; and the extent of client·involvement and responsibility in the situation. Any definition of competence for a profession must be related to an analysis of such factors in the total job situation. Shimberg (1977) reported that job analysis studies were being done in several professions to determine what practitioners actually did. Studies of critical incidents in physician performance were underscoring the necessity that physicians be able to integrate and apply their knowledge in problem-solving and decision-making situations. Hogan (1977) insisted that a delineation of potential outcomes was essential to an evaluation of competency, for without a clear picture of the possibilities there is no clarity about what the practitioner should be doing.

Pottinger (1977) found the classification of job requirements to be useful in identifying motor skills but too narrow for the more complex expectations of professional practice. He also rejected the behavioral objectives model where competence was tied to externally observed behaviors that may correlate with but not cause success. He believed the technique of behavioral events analysis—a structured interview involving the obtaining of descriptions of behavioral episodes—elicits information from which actual overt and covert behavior, which are in turn causally related to competent professional behavior, can be reconstructed.

McClelland and Boyatzis (1980) described a five-step behavioral events analysis process which led to the definition and operationalization of job-related competency and which was tied to outcome. They focus, in this example, on the U.S. Navy alcoholism counselors. First, they identified some outstanding and average performers in a position by asking persons who knew the job to generate a list of superior performers. Second, behavioral events interviews were conducted which focused on the actions, thoughts, and feelings involved in vividly successful or unsuccessful recent job events to gain a picture of how outstanding and average performers go about doing their jobs. The third step was to conceptualize competencies emerging from this data collection that differentiated superior from average performers and that were stated in terms that permitted them to become operational. In the case of the outstanding U.S. Navy alcoholism counselors, these competencies included: (1) a greater sense of personal power and impact, (2) a greater ability to think in terms of causal patterns in a patient's behavior, (3) more sensitivity to patient's verbal and nonverbal cues, (4) more awareness of personal feelings in the counseling situation, and (5) a greater desire for personal growth. Following the conceptualization step, the fourth step was to find or develop measures for these competencies that differentiated between the two groups. The fifth and final step was to administer the measures to a different group of individuals in the position for whom there are also job performance measures to see the extent to which they differentiate the outstanding from the average performers. In the case of the alcoholism counselors, four of the five competencies actually differentiated the outstanding from the average counselors. Eleven of the fifteen outstanding counselors had four or more of the competencies in a high degree while only two of fourteen average counselors had them in high degree. Eighty-seven percent of the alcoholic counselees of the outstanding counselors returned to duty and had satisfactory work performance ratings while only 70 percent of the counselees of the average counselors did the same. In this study they were not able to successfully operationalize the final criterion, "desire for personal growth."

McGaghie (1980) described the Professional Performance Situation Model as it was applied to the profession of medical technology. Though there was no empirical reference to outstanding or minimal quality performance, it illustrated a procedure that "encourages evaluators to map key dimensions of professional behavior, thought, and the circumstances in which they occur . . . into a complex yet finite competence domain" (p. 306).

First, situation facets (general variables or features) were identified for medical technologists based on observations and expert reports. These facets were expected to be independent of one another, though when considering complex professions this criterion may not be satisfied. Five facets were identified: "(a) diagnostic analyses, (b) follow-up / monitoring analyses, (c) laboratory settings, (d) patient age, (e) clinical findings" (p. 307).

Second, the particular elements involved in each facet were identified (for example, the types of diagnostic analyses) and then ordered according to frequency of occurrence. This led to the third step, which was to construct from these elements a situations universe. Multiplying thirty analyses by five follow-up procedures, by nine settings, by five age groups, and by four types of findings results in 27,000 situations, a large but finite number of situations with a known structure. "The universe provides an unambiguous operational description of the professional domain of medical technology"

(p. 308). From this universe, the fourth step was to systematically draw a sample of eighteen medical technology situations.

Since the eighteen situations did not include a description of skill and knowledge requirements, the fifth step had four experienced medical technologists, supervised by the researchers, write brief scenarios which included descriptions of what was supposed to happen when a medical technologist encountered each situation. The scenarios were then analyzed in a sixth step to determine some 100 specific skill and knowledge components for each scenario.

The seventh and final stage of this investigation combined the specific knowledge and skill components into thirty-five statements of proficiency appropriate to entry-level medical technologists.

Though empirical work was done to establish validity and measurement capability, space limitations preclude the inclusion here of the procedures. The importance of this work, however, is its contribution to systematically identifying the "dimensions and interrelationships of relevant professional content" (p. 310) so that the situations in which practice occurs can be inserted into the competency equation.

Procedures that similarly relate the significant characteristics of the person to critical aspects of the situation are necessary if competency assessment is to develop valid information about human performance in sensitive service occupations. Since the manner in which competency is measured becomes the operational definition of the competency, several writers have paid attention to the characteristics of measurement that lead to more valid assessments of competency. Referring to her experience in developing a training program for human service professionals, Goldsmith (1979) wrote:

Ideally, competency assessment is an approach that: evaluates performance rather than information mastery; judges ability rather than achievement; measures what can be demonstrated in the world rather than verbal descriptions about what can be demonstrated; evaluates active participation rather than passive analysis; and brings us closer to knowing if the professional has the ability to make a positive impact on clients. [p. 54]

McClelland (1973) suggested five criteria to use in judging the adequacy of assessment procedures. In the main, these criteria help assessment strategies emerge that focus less on what people *bring* to practice and more on what they *do* with what capabilities they have.

1. *Assessment is criterion referenced.* Assessment in a particular occupation is based on successful performance in practice rather than a general intelligence factor and specified performance standards rather than comparisons (norm referenced) between persons being assessed. The behavioral events analysis previously described is one example of the application of this first criterion for assessment. Measures need not be paper and pencil standardized tests. The "assessment

center" approach permits measurement of behavior in situations similar to those faced day to day.

2. *Assessment is reflective of participant's growth.* Rather than seek unmodifiable characteristics as proxies for an operationalized competency, assessment should be designed to identify characteristics that respond to learning. Such assessment is more likely to be valid if people are able to show better performance as the result of training and experience.

3. *Assessment criteria are public and explicit.* Rather than be concerned about keeping the public ignorant of the assessment material and criterion, they should be open to public viewing and clearly relevant to performance. Concern about participants "faking" an ability they do not have is reduced when there is a connection between the ability being assessed and the desired performance. For example, one cannot fake a road test of the ability to drive a vehicle. The alternative to openness is the game psychologists have been playing with participants over the secrecy of test answers.

4. *Assessment focuses on competencies involved in clusters of life outcomes.* Rather than assess a large number of highly specific skills involved in performance, assessment should center on more general underlying competencies that differentiate successful and unsuccessful practitioners. McClelland (1973) identified communication skills, patience, moderate goal setting, and ego development as such personal competencies. By so doing, he avoids considering the plethora of skills that may correlate with but are not causally related to competence.

5. *Assessment emphasizes spontaneous responses.* Rather than depending upon situation-structured responses where the stimulus is designed to evoke a specific response, assessment should involve an operant type of response, more typical of the kind of decision making in everyday life where individuals respond spontaneously in the absence of very clearly defined cues. In this regard, Klemp (1979) suggested that the criterion of correctness of response be replaced by the criterion of effectiveness, where more than one response is appropriate. Because the emphasis is on spontaneity in responding, the participant is less likely to give the same responses in successive assessments, thereby raising questions about reliability. New ways of viewing reliability may have to be developed to suit this type of assessment.

The issue of determining competency is, indeed, a complex one. Since traditionally defined qualifications have not been found to ensure competency, new approaches are required for any system, whether public or private, that would credential practitioners. The goal of developing performance-based examinations that rely on criteria validated on client outcomes appears to be beyond the state of the art at this time for most professional and occupational categories. The developments are such, however, to suggest that this circumstance is more related to the lack of incentives than to the impossibility of the task. If, however, it is decided that it is impossible to validly estimate practitioner competence this would turn into another argument against the advisability of attempting to protect consumers and for information-based strategies that would enhance consumer self-protection.

8

LICENSURE AND QUALITY

The generally stated purpose for licensing and the primary justification for this use of the police power of the State is to ensure quality in the services offered to the public. Until recently, the relationship between licensing and quality was rarely questioned; it appeared so self-evident that if one conscientiously restricts entry into a profession the result will be that the better practitioners survive the entry process. The contemporary critique of the professions has questioned this conventional wisdom and served to stimulate a steady stream of investigations on this topic in the last decade. The problems of defining and measuring quality are being approached seriously.

Defining quality does pose complex problems of clarification and measurement. Begun (1980) indicated that the use of the word *quality* may refer to "the degree of respect for the professional, the degree of communication or humanism in the professional-client relation, the technical sophistication of the service, or the actual outcome of the service" (p. 10).

Given such variation, it is important to be specific about how the word *quality* is being used and in what context. Typically quality measures are described in three ways: as *structural* or inputs into services, such as provider's educational level or technical competence; as measures of the *process* or the procedures involved in providing services, such as the patient-provider relationship; and as measures of *outcome* of the services provided, such as the reduction of problematic symptoms in a population. There may be variation in how well these measures are specified and how well they relate to the phenomenon being measured. For example, holding a B.A. degree would concretely describe a candidate's educational level without indicating qualifications to perform a particular task.

The question of what purpose the standard of quality is to serve is also important. Should quality standards establish a minimal floor of acceptable practice, a high standard of practice, or should they reflect the current practice in a profession?

The critical practical question is, however, *who* should define "quality?" Researchers and consumers tend to prefer outcome measures, reasoning that the consequences of a service are what matter in the long run. Professionals have preferred process measures as these measures lend themselves most easily to peer monitoring and permit professionals themselves to contol the determination of quality for society as a whole. By so doing, however, they have tended to ignore such input measures as measures of availability of service and outcome measures generally. For example, Spiegel and Backhaut (1980) indicated that the quality of health care was directly linked with five characteristics of its delivery system: the extent to which the service was actually made available; if available, the extent to which it was accessible to patients; if accessible, the extent to which it was acceptable to patients; and, if acceptable, the extent to which it was provided with continuity, and at an affordable cost. These have not been important concerns for professionals.

The traditional approach of professionals has been to maintain quality through licensing, ethical codes, and other restraints on competition. Blair and Kaserman (1980) found a "curious form of social contract" to result.

In essence, the professionals as a group have decided that one motivation for reducing the quality of the services provided by individual members is the lure of higher income. As a result, the profession guards against that quality deterioration by reducing competition and raising the average income level of its members. In effect, society pays a bribe in the form of noncompetitive fees and then hopes that this will prevent low-quality services. [p. 185]

Hamilton (1982) believed that through these practices by professions a myth of perfection was perpetrated as a standard of quality that resulted in few choices available to consumers of health care. She argued that "Quality does not mean perfection; neither must it mean the same services by the same kind of providers. Instead, it is a range of acceptable variance in relation to the price charged" (p. 62). Hamilton's evaluation criticized outcome measures as they are influenced by social, environmental, and hereditary factors that affect patient responses to treatment. On the other hand, the physician's art of care influences patient self-care, influencing, in turn, outcomes. Hamilton preferred structural measures that refer to the character of the institution in which care was delivered. Work settings have been found to be more influential as far as the quality of physician behavior is concerned than the physician's formal education.

Nicholas Cummings, former president of the American Psychological Association, announced an effort to enhance quality care called the 'National Academies of Practice" (1982). He acknowledged that this was not being done by professional associations. He announced that the first goal would be "to define quality of practice, then measure it. Do you know it's never been done?" (p. 2).

Milton Roemer's (1970) discussion of six basic conditions necessary for the achievement of high-quality medical care for a population included both process and outcome factors. He emphasized that all were subject to improvement via social action.

Maintain a safe and hygienic environment. This condition involves not only environmental factors that may contribute to death, disease, and disability, on one hand, or positive "wellness," on the other but also the practices of service givers to the extent that their procedures, equipment, and personnel enhance or negate favorable environments or decisions for consumers. This condition refers to the prevention efforts of governmental bodies, as well as professionals, in the control of negative factors and the development of positive factors.

Foster an educated public. This condition refers to the ability of the public to make decisions regarding life-style and the use of professional resources, both of which contribute to the level of quality. Education is crucial here in the sense that people require information and understanding to make necessary decisions.

Develop an adequate supply of physical and human resources. This condition refers to the extensiveness of the supply of personnel, facilities, and equipment pertinent to the adequacy of service delivery. Investment of financial resources and long term planning are involved in developments in this area.

Maintain financial access to resources. Whether available resources are accessed by a population is in part determined, in our society, by the availability of private funds or, increasingly, coverage under insurance laws or welfare legislation.

Maintain location and communication access to resources. Whether resources are accessed by a population is in part determined by the reasonable location of the resources and the corresponding distance or difficulty posed by transportation and communication systems and styles.

Maintain continuing flow of new knowledge. Social and economic support is concentrated on the development of new knowledge pertinent to the needs of the public, on the dissemination of knowledge to practitioners, and on enhancing the impact of knowledge on practice.

Roemer's (1970) review of these factors promoting quality in medical care concluded:

There is no sector of the field about which we can be satisfied. Relative to our scientific knowledge or the demonstrated achievements in particular plans, we can say that there are serious deficiencies in quality maintenance throughout the nation. Our potentialities for maintaining standards on personnel and facilities for sound institutional organization, for disciplinary incentives, and for continuing education, regionalization, and so on, are far greater than have been implemented in practice. [p. 300]

Roemer's (1970) criteria are obviously very general and might not apply equally to all professions. They obviously refer primarily to health occupations. To adjust them to other occupations, the reader should consider the purpose of the occupation. Applying this to lawyers, for example, we might want to change the first criterion to refer instead to the maintenance of social, political, and legal structures that enhance consumer rights and public security.

These definitions of quality are suggestive of the problems of monitoring quality. We now turn to our central concern in this chapter—probing the relationship between licensure and quality. First is an examination of how attempts to regulate professional service by input monitoring (for example, restrictions on entry) affect quality measures. Process monitoring for quality is discussed later in this chapter in the section on examining agency functioning. Other process measures such as self-regulation and output monitoring have been discussed in chapter 5. This chapter will conclude with a discussion of the role of licensing as a determiner of *poor* quality.

RESEARCH ON LICENSING AND QUALITY MEASURES

By preventing incompetent or unscrupulous providers from serving the public, legal restrictions on occupational entry are supposed to result in a higher quality of service to consumers than would occur in the absence of restriction.

In just the last few years a number of studies of licensing and quality service have been reported that offer somewhat contradictory results. They represent a beginning attempt to probe the question of quality and licensing but unfortunately do not provide profoundly credible results. Readers should bear in mind the prior disinterest in this area, the newness of this area of investigation, and the difficulties in operationalizing, measuring, and controlling variables to explain the relative crudeness of these studies and the inconsistencies between some of them.

Despite the conclusions of economic and sociological theorists about the financial and social costs of a monopolistic licensing system as well as questions about its effectiveness, much of the public and many professionals are either unaware of the cost or convinced that any cost is worth the price. Many are uncritical, believing that licensing protects the public. Though research is not often instrumental in influencing public policy, the illusion of protection and the belief that it is worth the price has been in part maintained by the lack of evidence on the protection issue and by the fact that recent evidence has not found its way out of the scholarly journals. The findings and conclusions of twenty-five research studies, most of which have been completed since 1977, have been compiled, bringing together the empirical research on licensing and quality.

Peer Ratings and Self-reports

Restriction on entry into an occupation is an attempt to limit the input into an occupation by removing low-quality service suppliers. Following this reasoning the relationship between restrictions on entry and quality of licensed practitioners should be positive; the more or higher the restrictions, the higher the quality. Three studies suggest this. Carroll and Gaston (1981a) found a positive relationship between quality and restrictiveness in their study of attorneys. Using a widely respected peer evaluation system as the quality offered measure, they found a positive relationship (significant at the .05 level of confidence) with a bar exam residency requirement (an entry restriction). A negative relationship (significant at the .01 level of confidence) between the peer measure and a measure of attorney density indicated that smaller numbers of attorneys were associated with higher quality of service offered. The authors did raise the question that professional cohesiveness may bias the peer-rating measure since their peer evaluation system rated highest those attorneys who came from smaller, nonurbanized states.

Holen's (1978) study focused on participation of dentists in continuing education. Her study was important for two reasons. First, the data were drawn from a survey conducted between 1966 and 1969 before any state mandated continuing education. Second, continuing education is believed by many to be a valid way to maintain quality in the services of autonomous professionals. Holen's analysis indicated that a significant positive association existed between fail rate (high restrictiveness) and percentage of dentists reporting continuing education courses. She did not report the significance level but concluded that "states that pass a small percentage of applicants in the licensing examination tend to select those who are more likely to participate in further professional education" (p. 23). The inference here was that their report of participation is a quality measure. When she attempted, however, to relate participation in continuing education to another quality measure (lower malpractice premiums) she got the expected negative association, but it was not statistically significant, thus raising a question about the relevance of the report of participation in continuing education as a measure of quality.

Begun (1980) did a questionnaire study of optometrists. His results supported the association between licensing and quality, though his 54 percent return on questionnaires did contain some nonresponse bias. His variable "legislated professionalism" included the extent to which the licensing laws of a state contained one or more of the following: required continuing education, Doctor of Optometry price advertising prohibited, optician advertising prohibited, mercantile location restricted. He used three process quality variables: examination length, examination complexity (number of specified procedures used), and office equipment (number of items available). He found a positive association between legislated professionalism and examination length significant at the .01 level. When compared, his licensing and the other two quality variables did not have a significant association. The required continuing education variable was significantly (P < .01) related to all three quality measures while mercantile location was significantly (P < .01) related to exam complexity and office equipment. Prohibiting price advertising, whether by optometrists or opticians, had no relationship to any of the quality measures. Respondents' self-report of continuing education hours was positively related (P < .01) to all three quality measures.

Client Reactions

Turning to a quality-received measure, client reactions should be more positive if licensing is working to enhance quality. Maurizi (1977a) compared consumer complaints for thirty-two licensing boards in California in relationship to a measure of restrictiveness (the pass rate on application). After dropping two boards because of potential errors in reporting frequency of complaints, he found the pass rate to be significantly *negatively* related to the number of complaints reported. In this case, high restrictiveness was associated with higher numbers of complaints. Maurizi, however, suggests caution about this result because assumptions essential to his analysis of the data were found to be inappropriate. In Maurizi's study of the Structural Pest Board (1977b), he found that the number of complaints per licensee declined when entry was less rstricted. This study was criticized by Harris (1978) for selecting a measure that biased the study toward accepting the hypotheses, so caution is advised here also.

In his study of contractors, Maurizi (1977c) was forced to reject his assumption that licensing boards were restricting competent people from the field. Instead, he found that the growth in the number of schools teaching contractors how to pass the exam explained the increased number of complaints because the exam did not screen out incompetent contractors. Maurizi's studies of complaints cannot be said to indicate a relationship between complaints and licensing, though he appears to be pioneering research in a promising direction.

In a study of consumer ratings, Muris and McChesney (1979) compared lawyers who advertised with those who did not. Since advertising is often prohibited by licensing statutes, it is used here as a substitute variable for licensing. An 11-percent return of a mailed survey of clients showed no significant differences between traditional firms (nonadvertisers) and a legal clinic (advertisers) on consumer ratings of promptness, concern, honesty, explanations, keeping client informed, and attending. Being fair and reasonable in fee charges showed a significantly superior rating for the clinic at the .03 level of confidence.

Malpractice insurance rates are a crude measure of quality received because they are affected by many factors, including willingness of attorneys to represent aggrieved clients, the size of damage awards, and statutory restrictions in size of awards. One study presented data relating entry restrictions to malpractice insurance rates. Holen (1978) did not find statistical significance, though she did report negative relationships between pass rates on entry examination (high restrictiveness) and low malpractice insurance rates for dentists. Carroll and Gaston (1981a), however, found a significant positive relationship between a peer measure of quality offered by attorneys and malpractice rates. These findings, however, are subject to the limitation noted earlier about peer ratings.

Formal disciplinary actions against attorneys are a crude measure of quality in that they too are subject to some of the limitations expressed earlier about malpractice claims and peer ratings. Carroll and Gaston (1981a) did find, however, that the higher the peer rating, the fewer the number of disciplinary actions. Since these peer ratings were related to restrictiveness, this result lends support to those associating licensing and quality.

Substitution Effects

Carroll and Gaston (1977) take what they call a broader view of quality by looking unobtrusively at quality *received* by consumers. Licensing is seen to create a substitution incentive for consumers in that they react to the fewer and more expensive providers by either utilizing unorthodox providers or "doing it themselves." (Those studies where consumers react by choosing a "no service" option and those where the service is simply less available, are reviewed in the section on availability effects.) In the instance where substitution occurs, Carroll and Gaston argue, a lower quality service results. There are studies of two occupations where the self-service measure was used.

In their study of plumbers, Carroll and Gaston (1977) used retail sales of plumbing supplies per household as the "do it yourself" measure. Density of plumbers was significantly negatively related to plumbing sales at the .05 level of confidence, but two tests of licensing restrictiveness were not significantly related to density. This suggested that unionization of plumbers was more of a factor in plumber density than licensing. In their study of electricians, Carroll and Gaston (1981b) used a rather macabre "do it yourself" measure—accidental death by electrocution. In this case, the licensing restrictive measures were significantly associated with density. Low density was negatively and significantly related to death by electrocution when they compared this data to the density of both journeymen and master electricians.

Availability

Availability measures assume that quality received is a function of the amount of service actually offered. Though Holen (1978) did not find evidence of a relationship between her measure of availability (the number of visits to dentists per capita) and a measure of restrictiveness (pass rate), she did associate positively her measure of availability with her quality measure (percentage of dentists reporting continuing education). She used this data to conclude that "more stringent licensing standards may be beneficial to consumers" (p. 38). On the other hand, Carroll and Gaston (1981b) found dentist density to be negatively associated (significant at the .01 level of confidence) with feelings by dentists that they were too busy (a low availability measure) and positively (significant at the .05 level of confidence) with feelings that they were not busy enough (a high availability measure). Long work weeks and long delays (low availability measures) were significantly related to high restrictions on numbers of dentists at the .05 and .01 levels of confidence, respectively. In their study of sanitarians, Carroll and Gaston (1977) associated availability with an absence of health inspections (inviting deterioration in public health services received). They found restrictive licensing to reduce the numbers of sanitarians in rural areas and the inner city but not in suburban areas or small towns.

Carroll and Gaston (1978) found veterinarian density in a state's population was positively and significantly related to the reported cases of rabies and brucellosis in animals. They indicated that there was a "systematic underdiscovering of existing cases" (p. 39) and a consquent risk to other animals and to people in states with low density of veterinarians. The restrictive devices in this case were the use of U.S. citizenship as an entry requirement and the limitation on the number and the enrollment in schools of veterinary medicine.

In the Carroll and Gaston (1979a) study of the real estate business, a "duration of vacancy prior to sale" rate was used as the quality variable. They concluded, "in states where overall numbers of brokers per capita are low, *urban* service quality suffers; [and] where either pass rates are depressed by licensing authorities or where there are specified prior educational requirements, the result is lower quality service in *rural* areas" (p. 10).

Direct Outcome

Holen (1978), using the presence of dental disease among naval recruits as a quality measure, found a nonsignificant, negative relationship with fail rate and interpreted this trend to relate stricter licensing to dental health. Nor did she find significance in the relationship between licensing and edentulousness (absence of teeth) as a measure of quality of dental care. Carroll and Gaston (1981b), using an oral hygiene index constructed by the Naval Medical Research Command, found that reciprocity (low restriction) increases density of dentists. Density was positively related to good oral hygiene. Reviewing census data, they also found "that the smaller numbers of dentists *per capita* are associated with more widespread tendencies among those who own false teeth to never wear them, indicating, perhaps, that the dentures, for whatever reason, are not satisfactory" (p. 16). Healey's (1973) study used a measure of clinical laboratory proficiency she believed had questionable validity. She compared proficiency data between laboratories in a state with restrictive licensing and a state that had no licensure restriction. She did not find personnel licensure to significantly improve the output quality of a laboratory.

Phelan's (1974) study of the television repair industry reported on the comparative incidence of fraud in three contrasting jurisdictions: one licensed (New Orleans), one registration jurisdiction that had unannounced investigations of television service dealers for fraud (San Francisco), and one that had no statutory entry restriction (Wahington, D.C.). "Parts fraud" is the unnecessary replacing of parts or charging for parts not actually replaced. Approximately twenty repair dealers in each location were given identically malfunctioning TV sets. Parts fraud occurred in 50 percent of the cases in both New Orleans (licensed) and Washington, D.C. (unlicensed), and only in 20 percent of the cases in San Francisco (registered investigations). Investigation activities rather than licensing appeared to influence parts fraud.

In a study done for the Federal Trade Commission (Bond et al., 1980), advertising of services by optometrists was related to several direct outcome measures of quality. Extent of restrictiveness on advertising is comparable to licensing as indicated previously because it is often associated with licensing. The results are suggestive. On a client-rating measure when nonadvertising optometrists were compared to advertisers, nonadvertisers were rated by clients as giving more thorough examinations. There was, however, no observed difference between advertisers and nonadvertisers on these outcome quality measures: obtaining the correct prescription and producing adequate eyeglasses, quality of workmanship of the eyeglasses, incidence of unnecessary prescription of eyeglasses, and quality of eye examinations.

A Muris and McChesney study (1979) of lawyers who did or did not advertise used as a direct outcome measure a multiple regression analysis of the influence on the amount of child-support awards. Better service when the client was the husband was defined as a lower award of child support and when the client was the wife, as a higher award. Husband's gross income and wife's expenses had expected positive effects on the size of the award, while number of children negatively affected the size of the award per child. Wife's gross income and husband's expenses did not affect the size of the award. The representation of the husband by lawyers who did not advertise had no statistically significant effect on the size of the award. When advertisers represented the wife, there was a significant ($p < .025$) positive effect on the size of the award. They concluded that firms that advertise did "not necessarily produce lower quality service" and that the "one clinic studied actually provides *better* quality than its traditional competitors" (pp. 205-6). The limitation here is that the study focusing on one firm is not necessarily generalizable. It is important, however, that the expected association between advertising and lowered quality did not occur.

Summary

The studies of the relationship between licensing and quality are certainly a confusing array of findings and conclusions (table 8.1). Readers should bear in mind the prior disinterest in this area, the newness of this area of investigation, and the difficulties in operationalizing, measuring, and controlling variables as explanation for the relative crudeness of and inconsistency between some of the studies. These studies represent an exciting opening of an area of investigation more than they represent observations on which policy may be based. Finally, it should be added that these are studies of association, therefore causation should not be presumed.

With these caveats, what can be said at this point? Removing the studies involving the questionable peer review procedure (Carroll and Gaston, 1981a), conflicting quality data (Holen, 1978), and assumptions and methods that the authors questioned (Healey, 1973; Maurizi, 1977a, 1977b, 1977c), two studies remain suggesting a positive association between licensing and quality (Begun, 1980; Bond et al., 1980). Begun's (1980) study is impressive because of the care he took in defining his criteria and in controlling his variables and design. Ignoring the facts that this is a self-report study with admitted nonresponse bias and involving process measures, his results do show some positive relationships between licensing and quality as he defines it. Optometrists in more restrictive states did spend more time with their patients. They, however, did not use more procedures or have more equipment available. In Bond et al. optometrists who did not advertise gave more thorough examinations than advertisers according to client investigators. There were, however, no other observed differences on direct outcome measures, including obtaining correct prescriptions and producing adequate eyeglasses. The positive connection, then, between licensing and measures of quality is not clearly established by these studies.

The remaining client reaction studies show no association (Holen, 1978; Muris and McChesney, 1979). Similarly, direct outcome studies primarily show no association (Bond et al., 1980; Holen, 1978; Muris and McChesney, 1979; Phelan, 1974).

Though Carroll and Gaston (1981b) found reciprocity, high density of

TABLE 8.1 Research Studies of Licensing and Quality of Service, according to Type of Quality Measure

Subject Evaluations and Reports	Client Reactions	Substitution Effects	Availability Effects	Outcome
Peer Ratings	*Complaints*	§Carroll and Gaston (1977)	‡Carroll and Gaston (1977)	§Bond et al. (1980)
*†Carroll and Gaston (1981a)	†‡Maurizi (1977a)	‡Carroll and Gaston (1981b)	‡Carroll and Gaston (1978)	‡Carroll and Gaston (1981b)
	†‡Maurizi (1977b)		‡Carroll and Gaston (1979a)	†§Healey (1973)
Self-report	†§Maurizi (1977c)		‡Carroll and Gaston (1981b)	§Holen (1978)
*†Holen (1978)			§Holen (1978)	§Muris and McChesney (1979)
*Begun (1980)	*Malpractice Claims*			§Phelan (1974)
	§Holen (1978)			
	*†Carroll and Gaston (1981a)			
	‡Martin (1980)			
	Disciplinary Proceedings			
	*†Carroll and Gaston (1981a)			
	Client Evaluations			
	*Bond et al. (1980)			
	§Muris and McChesney (1979)			

*Significant positive relationship found between licensing and quality.
†Questionable procedure or contradictory findings.
‡Significant negative relationship found between licensing and quality.
§No relationship found between licensing and quality.

dentists, and a measure of good oral hygiene to be associated, the most impressive findings are those Carroll and Gaston studies (1981b, 1977, 1978, 1979a), which show the presence of substitution and availability effects. These indicate a negative relationship between licensing and quality. In the two remaining studies in this area (Carroll and Gaston, 1977; Holen, 1978), substitution and availability effects were not demonstrated. Though substitution and availability effects indirectly complement the high quality of orthodox service providers when they are readily available, they also point to an undersupply of orthodox providers as a negative consequence of restriction on entry. Frech (1974) supported this point.

Under licensing, by preventing entry of those with lower qualification, the quality of care rendered by *licensed professionals* may rise, but consumer substitution of other services such as chiropractors, the advice of friends and self-treatment, plus provider substitution of lower-skilled personnel for expensive licensed individuals could result in lower quality of care actually received. [p. 121].

We are led to speculate on the possibility of a negative consequence for licensing but, before this is accepted, other ways of demonstrating the negative relationship must be found. Meanwhile, the most acceptable conclusion is still that no adequate relationship between licensing and quality has been demonstrated.

EXAMINING LICENSING AGENCY FUNCTIONING

If licensing agencies were doing their job there should be evidence of fulfilling five functions, according to Cohen and Miike (1974): effective initial assessment of competence, monitoring continuing competence, discipline of errant practitioners, facilitation of the distribution of licensed professionals to needy areas and persons, and utilization of allied professionals where such persons are more competent and less costly than professionals. Though licensing agencies mainly attempt to assess initial competence, we shall look at the other four first.

Continuing Competence

The primary means by which licensing agencies attempt to maintain continuing competence is through continuing education. The trend in the 1970s has been to go from voluntary to mandatory continuing education. Though continuing education has face validity, it is now being questioned as to its efficacy and relevance, as we have indicated in chapter 5.

Shimberg (1977) indicated that state licensing boards mandated continuing education as a requirement for relicensure, despite "the lack of evidence that continuing education is necessarily related to performance on the job" (p. 158). State legislatures appear to have no other acceptable response to the concern for continuing competency. Despite some resistance, "the convenience and political safeness of continuing education are leading more and more legislators to require it" (Continuing Education, 1979). Some things are done because they are "something to do" or because they avoid doing something else or because they fulfill some other function. For example, an Arizona state senator who is also a chiropractor has led the effort to drop mandatory continuing education requirements. It is his opinion that "Continuing education is one more way the professions protect themselves and restrain trade. In the chiropractic profession the association could not get everyone to join, but was able to use mandated continuing education to force practitioners to fund the association" (Arizona Senator, 1980, p. 7).

A more promising alternative for encouraging practitioners to keep up with their fields is called *periodic reassessment*. This has met with strong resistance from practitioners, however. The only use of reassessment has been for nongovernmental recertification.

Discipline

Licensing does not seem to be effective in preventing incompetent practice. Lieberman (1970) reviewed studies of medical practice and surgery and found that "professional incompetence is nearing epidemic proportions in some areas" (p. 104). Looking at his own profession, he stated, "Cases of lawyers who continue to practice in spite of unethical conduct directly related to the lawyer's function are legion" (p. 105). Milgrom (1978) reviewed several studies of dental competency. In one, "only 63 percent of the newly placed amalgams observed were satisfactory . . . two percent needed *immediate* replacement . . . (35 percent) had sufficient defects to require continued observation" (p. 6). Two other studies involving over 6,000 patients showed faulty amalgams in 44 and 45 percent of the cases. The importance of the numbers of patients affected is shown by the report in that one group of dentists studied replaced 6.6 amalgam surfaces each working day.

In the case of medicine, there is little interest in the discipline of incompetent practitioners. Derbyshire (1979), a former president of the Federation of State Medical Boards, has studied the problem of discipline for some time and stated that, despite his estimate that 5 percent of America's doctors are unfit to practice, only twenty-six states specify professional incompetence as a reason for disciplinary action. Hogan's (1979b) review of psychology legislation showed that, as a basis for discipline, only four states specifically cited incompetence, ten states cited practice outside area of competence, twenty-three states cited negligence, and only nineteen cited mental illness. Alcoholism and drug addiction were the leading personal disqualifiers cited in the laws of forty-four states. Milgrom (1978) found that dental boards generally imposed discipline for reasons having to do with advertising, conviction for a criminal offense, substance abuse, unsanitary conditions, and such vague terms as physical or mental incapacity and professional misconduct. He concluded, "Though few would challenge the fact that these are serious conditions and no doubt affect the quality of care a dentist provides, they are very indirect reflections of that quality" (p. 117).

In general, boards tend to be more zealous in prosecuting unlicensed practitioners than in disciplining those already licensed. Hogan (1979a) found that complaints against the unlicensed brought by licensed personnel tended to increase in one study when economic conditions worsened. Table 8.2 describes the experience of one licensing agency that received comparatively few complaints. Forty percent of the complaints related to practice without a license. Summerfield (1978) believed that what he judged to be an "incredibly" small number of complaints was caused by patients who did not know where to complain (the Psychology Examining Committee was not even listed in city telephone books in California) and by those who did not want the stigma connected with being "mental" patients to reflect on their personal adequacy. With regard to this stigma, McKinlay and Dutton (1974) discussed the effect of labeling persons as "mentally ill," "alcoholic," "obese," and so on. Once so labeled, a person is potentially "discreditable." Fearing that, many people do not complain about inadequate service to avoid the public application of the label.

The political nature of the problem of discipline is revealed by the contrasting view of the action of the state boards as expressed in the use of the differing modifiers italicized below. Derbyshire (1969) conducted two studies of state board disciplinary actions. Referring to the first study, his material was vague about the actual number of incompetents, but of the 1,000 disciplinary actions taken over a five-year period, he said *many* were because of incompetence. Shryock (1967) referring to Derbyshiire's first study, thought the number was *not large*. He wondered how effective the board actions were but concluded that "the medical members of the boards were making *some* effort at professional self-discipline in the public interest" (p. 114, emphasis added). Cohen (1973), on the other hand, referring to Derbyshire's latter study of 938 board actions over a four-year period said "*only* 400 were based upon some form of incompetence" (p. 3, emphasis added). Carlson (1976) discovered Derbyshire's (1974) updating of studies of medical discipline covering the years 1968 through 1972, indicating that 1,034 disciplinary actions were taken. When these were "combined with his earlier findings, one in 1,500 physicians had been disciplined by state licensure boards in each of the years studied" (p. 249). Carlson (1976) concluded,

. . . the most important point, however, is not evident from the data. Since the grounds for action against a physician under licensure statutes only rarely, if ever, go to the question of the performance by that physician in the duties for which he or she was trained, the actions taken by licensure boards against physicians are related to quality only in the most indirect sense. [p. 249]

TABLE 8.2 Open Cases (as of March 1978) of Complaints Made to California's Psychology Examining Committee, according to Violation and Determination of Whether Patient Abuse Was Involved (Cases Originating in 1975, 1976, and 1977)

Violation	Case Involved Patient Abuse	Case Did Not Involve Patient Abuse
Functioning outside area of competence	0	0
Unsound interpersonal relations	12	3
Misrepresentation of qualifications	0	1
Leaks confidential information	4	2
Fails to maintain test security	1	0
Fails to maintain professional identification	0	0
No PEC approval of assistants	0	0
Practice without a license	27	101
Assistant practicing without a license	0	0
Conviction for a felony or moral turpitude	6	12
Use of narcotics or abuse of alcohol	0	0
Impersonating a licensee	0	1
Application fraud	0	2
Fee splitting	0	0
Grossly negligent	11	8
Violates provision of code	7	14
Excessive treatment	15	11
Abets unlawful practice	0	6
Ethics or fee	2	14
Other	3	24
Total	88	199

Source: H. L. Summerfield, *Review of Psychology Examining Committee and State Board of Behavioral Science Examiners: A Report of the Regulatory Review Task Force* (State of California, Department of Consumer Affairs, 1978), pp. I-35–I-38.

Derbyshire (1979) recently reviewed the problem of physician competence and reported that the profession was beginning to recognize it as a real problem but was not squarely facing it. In the ten years from 1969 to 1979, the number of states specifying incompetence as cause for disciplinary action more than doubled, from twelve to twenty-six, but the charge was rarely invoked. Of the 1,768 disciplinary actions reported to the Federation of State Medical Boards between 1974 and 1977 only 48 were for incompetence. This represented 2.7 percent of the disciplinary actions but .24 percent of his estimate of 20,000 incompetent physicians then in practice. Very little improvement occurred for the estimated ten million Americans treated by these physicians annually. Derbyshire had hope for "sick doctor" laws and laws requiring physicians to report incompetent colleagues. Though he also had hope for the Joint Commission on the Accreditation of Hospitals' required annual physician reviews and professional review activities, he rated some of these approaches as "commendable if not yet fully effective, while those of others rate from poor to zero" (p. 103).

Krause (1977) reviewed studies of discipline and found little policing of peers "even in cases of extreme malfeasance" (p. 284). Since physicians are autonomous, they can and do determine the extent to which professional incompetence is defined as a social problem. The lack of action on this problem indicates that is to their self-interest to obscure the problem. Lieberman (1970) explained that the reputation of a profession was involved, therefore, there was activity in those areas relevant to the public image of the profession but little where image was not involved.

The theory of discipline is also tied to the public image of the professionals. . . . In fact, discipline is for any unorthodoxy of a public nature. . . . When the public does not know about the misdeeds of one of their fellows, there is no need to act since that would only call attention to it. Nor is there reason to disbar or eject a member permanently if the public is likely to forget. [pp. 108-9]

Board staffs, according to Cohen (1973), were ordinarily inadequate to carry out investigations, and the statutory provisions for such investigations were often marked by ambiguity and a lack of precision. One new licensing watchdog agency in the District of Columbia, specifically set up to reduce physician abuse, despite sweeping powers, could not keep pace with the complaints (Efforts, 1978). Even with the legal authority, lack of funds and staff are the reason the director's message to the public was "you're not protected here" (p. 3). The comprehensive legal study by Grad and Marti (1979) found that medical boards suffer, as far as disciplinary proceedings are concerned, from inadequate staffs, insufficient budgets, part-time board members, and inadequate records, if records are kept at all. In a nine-state survey they were often told that running a licensing program left little time for anything else, including managing a discipline program. All of this accounted for "the minimal record of accomplishment in investigating and following up complaints and in dealing with disciplinary matters" (pp. 22-23). The study by Arkansas Consumer Research (Clemons et al., 1981) is a case in point.

Responses to an ACR survey by 113 boards [out of 175] indicate that one third of the boards do not investigate complaints against service providers. . . . [A] lackadaisical attitude about enforcement responsibilities . . . is not solely the fault of the boards. By law, disciplinary options available to boards are limited. Enabling laws usually empower boards to suspend and revoke licenses, but the laws don't specify authority to utilize lesser methods.

Only a handful of boards explicitly have power to impose less than severe sanctions. [p. 39]

They concluded that the boards with more options can be more effective enforcers than those that have only severe sanctions available since they need not overlook less than severe transgressions. Many of these boards were also remiss in record keeping with only 27 out of 113 having records about complaints in 1979. Only sixty-seven of the board phone numbers could be found in the phone book for the state capital at Little Rock. With regard to public notice, twenty-five boards said they did not believe they had to provide public notice of meetings, while only twenty-nine reported that they did so.

Since licensing boards mostly respond to complaints rather than pursue their own investigations and since there is only a remote chance that any substantial penalty will be imposed, there is no support for the claim that licensing agencies hold practitioners accountable to high ethical standards. Cohen and Miike (1974) explained that the ineffectiveness of licensing boards is based on four factors:

a) There is a natural reluctance on the part of board members to invoke disciplinary action against their fellow practitioners;

b) disciplinary actions often result in lawsuits against the boards thereby causing boards to drop certain actions if an adverse ruling by the courts is anticipated;

c) board members function both as rule makers and rule adjudicators in deciding disciplinary matters, thereby causing confusion and overlap of roles; and

d) statutory provisions delineating the grounds for board sanctions generally are ambiguous, leading to judicial reluctance to enforce them. [p. 267]

Summerfield's (1978) review of California's system of regulating psychotherapy concluded, "The existing system seems quite close to the practitioner's ideal" (p. I-25). It is as Shimberg (1977) quipped, "Once licensed, forever competent" (p. 155). Hogan (1979a) concluded, "The formal disciplinary mechanism exercised by the state is not a significant factor in bringing about adherence to ethical norms and in ensuring minimal competency" (p. 261).

Maldistribution and Underutilization of Allied Professionals

Shortages of licensed personnel and underutilization of allied personnel are problems that are rarely considered by licensing agencies. These are problems to which licensing makes a contribution. The geographical maldistribution of professionals discriminated against "the elderly, the geographically isolated, the urban poor, the migrant workers" (National, 1967).

In an economic sense mobility is a mechanism by which the labor supply adjusts to changing conditions of demand. For individuals, mobility is one way to advance toward a career goal or to choose a better job. The flexible use of human resources to meet societal needs for service would require the free movement of practitioners from one location to another. The extent to which licensing puts up artificial restraints on mobility has a negative effect on the ability of occupations to respond to service needs, thus it negatively affects the quality received by the public.

Three studies show the effects professional licensing arrangements have on interstate mobility. Holen (1965) used 1950 census data and a 23-state, 1949 survey of medical, legal and dental income. Though she did not take note of actual reciprocity arrangements she presents evidence of interstate mobility in medicine, law and dentistry. She concluded, "Empirical evidence is consistent with the hypothesis that professional licensing arrangements and practices in dentistry and law restrict interstate mobility among dentists and lawyers and distort the allocation of professional personnel in these fields" (p. 498). Benham, Maurizi and Reder (1968) compared physicians and dentists on the consequences of barriers to migration. They found physicians tended to move where demand and income were high while interstate movement by dentists was impeded by state licensure arrangements.

Pashigian (1980) compared 24 occupations and concluded that the most pronounced effect of licensing is the reduced interstate mobility of members in licensed occupations. Restrictions on the use of reciprocity reduce interstate mobility still more. While licensed occupations have about the same within-state mobility as unlicensed occupations, they have significantly lower interstate migration rates. The evidence suggests that licensing is the primary reason for this difference. Licensing also appears to reduce the interstate mobility rates of older members more than it reduces that of younger workers. (pp. 326-28)

Roemer (1970) reported that, because of the concentration of medical practitioners, patients living in less populated areas were required to travel to distant medical centers for treatment. The likelihood of such travel depended on the patient's socioeconomic status. Milgrom (1978), a dentist himself, admitted: "Of course, the distribution of dentists *is* uneven. Like others, dentists choose to live and work in certain kinds of areas: they are frequently so crowded into affluent areas that they are entirely absent from central cities and rural areas" (p. 71).

Hogan's (1979a) review of the effect of licensing on the utilization of paraprofessionals indicated that licensing has had a profoundly negative effect. "By defining in extremely broad terms the practices restricted to fully licensed practitioners, and by making no provision or very rigid or narrow provisions for delegating functions to others, licensing laws unnecessarily limit those who can provide auxiliary services" (p. 277). The limitations restrict the number of paraprofessionals available to practice as well as their functioning on the job. They are prevented from performing many tasks of which they are capable either because of exclusionary language in licensing statutes or because fully licensed practitioners (for example, physicians) fear violating the law or malpractice suits in the absence of specific permission to delegate functions.

Summing up, Roemer (1970) considered the effectiveness of state licensure laws on minimal standards of competence.

Numerous questions can be raised about the effect of the state licensure laws in inhibiting free movement of health practitioners between states (in the interest of reducing professional competition within a state), thereby limiting quantitative resources in certain jurisdictions. There are also serious questions about the constraints against innovation in the laws governing licensure of nurses and other paramedical disciplines, which have special importance in coping with the increasing demands for medical care that cannot be met by our supply of doctors. [p. 287]

Initial Competence

The method by which licensing agencies assess initial competence is to evaluate the characteristics and abilities of candidates. Four types of qualifications are examined: personal characteristics such as age, citizenship, and residency in the jurisdiction; educational credentials; work experience such as internships or supervised practice; and results of written and oral examinations.

The definition of competency and how to evaluate it are controversial issues (see Chapter 7). Theoretical problems of clarifying the nature of competency (Koocher, 1979) are confused by political factors. Altering operational definitions of competency, no matter how faulty, could alter the existing division of labor or the dominance of certain groups. Haley (1975) reported the disruption occurring in a mental health facility upon the introduction of family therapy. As a method, Haley concluded, family therapy was incongruent with the medical model, hierarchical organization. There is a "shift in the status of the professions which comes about . . . [when] all the professions do the same work. . . . No profession has any more knowledge or training in family therapy than any other, and so the status hierarchy dissolves without a new one to take its place" (p. 10).

Using examples from the field of psychology, differences in income received by psychotherapists in mental health facilities, for example, were attributable to whichever of Tennov's (1975) seven academic credential routes were taken to qualify for the position (psychology, psychiatry, psychoanalysis, social work, clergy, nursing, or education), yet "distinctions . . . tend to be fictional since psychotherapists from different professions practice in much the same way" (p. 123) and even differences among schools of psychotherapy were negligible (Smith and Glass, 1977).

Summerfield (1978) also discounted the superiority of one training route over another. Instead he found that "Poor practice in psychotherapy may frequently be the result of the therapist's own inability to understand and to relate to his patients. That is, the psychotherapist's own personality is the principal tool of the treatment and the personality limitations of the therapist may be translated into clinical errors," (p. I-5).

Similarly, such requirements as citizenship, local residence, and good moral character have little relevance if one is estimating competence. Nonetheless, Milgrom (1978) cited evidence showing discrimination against out-of-state applicants for dental licenses. The state of Washington in 1975 failed 51 percent of out-of-state applicants but only 9.3 percent of in-state applicants.

Licensing agencies operationalize competency measures on the basis of what can be measured easily despite the lack of empirical validation. Consider Pottinger's (1977) report that the sheer amount of knowledge of a content area "is generally unrelated to superior performance in an occupation . . . [or] even to minimally acceptable performance" (p. 8), yet knowledge of content is predominantly what is measured in the multiple-choice format of written licensing exams.

A new development in testing are the "truth in testing" laws in California and New York State. They require publishers and users of tests to make available to examinees their completed test papers or a copy with correct answers noted. The need for legislation is a comment on the state of the art and the inadequacy of practice. It was Pottinger's (1979b) judgment that

Professions vary greatly in the quality of tests being used, but there are too many instances of certification tests that are poorly designed, constructed, validated and interpreted. The wide use of shoddy tests and the lack of accountability to test-takers in many occupations invites regulation of all certifying agencies not just those whose practices warrant it. [p. 8]

Hogan (1979a) found work experience to be an excellent predictor of competence. In psychology, Parloff (1979) found that though the "therapist's experience is related to the quality of the relationship . . . evidence regarding its association with outcome is far less clear" (p. 300). Knowing that more experienced people are more competent is not a sufficient guideline for licensing, yet numbers of years' experience are what one finds in licensing statutes (Hogan, 1979b).

Similarly, academic credentials are universally required, yet training does not identify the competent psychotherapist, for example (Hogan 1979a; Parloff, 1979), nor are grades or degrees found to be related to professional accomplishment generally (Collins, 1979). Shimberg (1982) reviewed studies that compared dentists with persons receiving as little as seven weeks of training in common dental procedures. Little or no differences were found. The comparable psychotherapeutic effectiveness often reported for para-professionals and lay persons who were trained on the job raises a great deal of doubt about the importance of theoretical and technical knowledge for minimal level competency (Hogan, 1979a; Parloff, 1979). Professional psychologists are also no more able when it comes to certain types of psychological diagnostic activity. Hogan (1979a) discussed the serious reliability and validity problems involved in such diagnostic activity. He indicated that for making gross distinctions (differentiating those who are mentally ill from those who are not) some paraprofessionals and patients were superior to professionals. Academic training is compromised as a basis for restricting entry if outcome measures (such as psychotherapeutic effectiveness and diagnostic accuracy) indicate such training makes no difference. This line of reasoning suggests that nonacademic routes to competence be recognized and that the assessment of competence relate directly to performance and practice.

Hogan (1979a) concluded from self-report surveys that clinical psychologists believe their training did not prepare them for clinical practice. The research orientations and antipractitioner attitudes in many academic departments were criticized in these surveys. The research of Henry et al. (1971) shows clinical psychologists to be significantly less satisfied with the value of their formal training than psychiatrists, psychoanalysts, and social workers were because this training emphasized an academic-research tradition at the expense of clinical experience. There is little reason to believe that input assessment of candidates for licensing in psychology has anything to do with the assessment of competence. Koocher (1979) concluded "that whatever existing credentials in psychology do measure they are clearly not highly valid measures of professional competence" (p. 702).

Mechanic (1979) took a similar position when viewing academic training in medicine.

. . . the effectiveness of long medical training as a screening device is an illusion. While medical schools attract applicants with a high level of academic competence, retention rates are extraordinarily high compared with most other types of graduate or postgraduate training and ensure little "weeding out" of undesirable candidates. Similarly, although supervision and negative appraisal during internship or residency may affect the ability of the candidate to obtain the most desirable positions, such supervision and evaluation almost never exclude the candidate from medical employment. In short, the image of a highly selective screening process that ensures quality and ethicality is a mirage, protecting the autonomy of the professional more than the public. [pp. 108-9]

In summary, it has been shown that licensing agencies do not function to protect life and property. Assessment of initial competence relies on invalid criteria. The monitoring of continued competence has not progressed beyond the questionable mandating of continuing education. Discipline of errant practitioners is confined mostly to prosecuting unlicensed practitioners rather than those already licensed. Licensing is seen as creating rather than ameliorating the problems of distribution of professionals and the utilization of paraprofessionals. The costs of licensing are not justified.

LICENSING AND INCOMPETENCE

So far, we have addressed the question of whether licensing fulfills its function to protect the public and concluded that competency is not enhanced and incompetency is not eliminated. In this section we turn the question around and ask: Is there a negative effect of licensing on the delivery of service? Is it merely irrelevant (aside from the costs detailed earlier) or does it provide a special haven for the incompetent or increase the likelihood that incompetent service will be delivered?

Some psychologists have been deeply concerned about the negative influence of licensing on psychologists themselves and have compared the products of the licensed and the unlicensed. Many psychologists may believe that Carl Rogers (1973) overstated the case when he said, "There are as many *certified* charlatans and exploiters of people as there are uncertified" (p. 382). Yet there is a strong support for Rogers's position. Tennov (1975) estimated that the damage done by untrained persons may be lower than that done by credentialed psychotherapists. Though acknowledging the warning that psychotic episodes can be precipitated by those who do not know what they are doing, Tennov believed that the tremendous authority given to the trained and licensed psychotherapist "makes it more likely that if harm is to be done, it will be he who does it" (p. 140). Hartley et al. (1976) and Hogan (1979a) reviewed studies that failed to show different levels of damage or deterioration effects for the conventional therapies as compared to the encounter therapies, which are more likely to be led by uncredentialed persons. Turning to medicine, Carlson (1976) indicated that the situation was no different when traditional medicine and other healing therapies were compared. When the "right" question was asked—that is, where patient outcome variables were more important than whether the practitioner used accepted tools and techniques in the treatment—there was no evidence that alternative therapies compromised the general quality of care.

Finally—though Cohen (1979) was rather deprecating about unlicensed psychotherapists, describing them as "uneducated, uncredentialed and unethical"—he concluded, "Unfortunately the good name of professional therapists is as likely to be sullied by an incompetent, non-credentialed 'therapist' as by a fellow professional" (p. 22). This was the result of many psychotherapists' unfounded belief that they could handle anyone who walked in the door. Greed and omnipotence played a part so that". . . even "legitimate" mental health professionals—such as licensed psychologists and board-certified psychiatrists—are not necessarily competent to render the services they offer to the public, owing to wide disparities in training backgrounds and inadequacies in formal credentialing procedures" (p. 261).

How it is possible that licensing arrangements could be implicated in encouraging professional incompetence? Licensing statutes may structure circumstances so that the net effect is increased danger to or exploitation of the public. The discussion refers mostly to the medical profession, but six factors are identified.

First, as we have shown, the rigidity of licensing laws in stipulating what can or cannot be done locks physicians into performing tasks, some of which could be performed more capably by an aide. Physicians are sometimes placed in the untenable position of being responsible for the performance of those who have superior knowledge and skill in areas in which the physician has little or no training. The rigidity of definition also tends to create an inertia that prolongs the use of orthodox but questionable treatments and delays the introduction of unorthodox but useful treatments.

Second, the dependency and mystification of the public, often encouraged by physicians, have created unrealistic expectations for what doctors are able to accomplish. Naive or dependent patients may ignore or delay acting on something that appears wrong, believing that the "doctor" will eventually rescue them. On the other hand, patients may fail to ask questions and will accept treatments, procedures, and medications not in their best interest because they believe the physician knows better than they do. The dangers of supposedly safe medications, the prevalence of unnecessary surgery, the overreadiness of physicians to prescribe inappropriate or dangerous drugs or use risky diagnostic procedures, and the failure of the public to mount significant objections have led social critic Ivan Illich (1976) to hypothesize a connection between the mystification and dependency of the public and iatrogenic effects. Cummings (1979) faults the medical model for inadvertently encouraging substance abuse by substituting one drug for another (methodone for heroin or valium for alcohol), a type of "addictive musical chairs" (p. 120). Likewise, Milgrom (1978) faulted dentists who, because of naivete about drugs, contributed to patients' shopping around for drugs by making pain medication available following telephone consultations, by keeping poor records, and by using prepared prescription forms provided by drug manufacturers. By promising but failing to protect the public, licensing systems increase the likelihood of iatrogenic effects because of the direct support given to continued public ignorance and trust.

Third, a physician's license to practice is too broad, certainly broader than most doctors' competency. Unfortunately, the desire for wealth and power have played a part in some physicians performing services for which they have little or no training. A recent study, for example, showed that 60 percent of identified mental patients were being treated by physicians who had little training in psychiatry (Parloff, 1979). Professional imperialism operates so as to broaden the scope of medicine to include treatments as practices for which the medical model has little relevance (for example, acupuncture).

Fourth, a credentials mentality exists that puts more stress on where and how people were trained than on what they can do. Ignoring productivity measures, the emphasis is more that treatment be accomplished in an approved, supposedly scientific manner. So-called scientific medicine rests, however, in a recent estimate, on procedures only 10 to 20 percent of which have been shown to be of benefit by controlled clinical trials (Office, 1978). The widespread disinterest in outcome cannot help but affect the actual quality of service delivered. Licensing is directly implicated here because it is the expression of the credentials mentality, the symbol of a way of thinking that emphasizes form over substance. Similarly, persons who fit the system are encouraged without regard to competence as Challes (1979) stated:

The system supports those who are technologically oriented or scientifically oriented while students who are people oriented and humanistically oriented have a hard time getting in or making it through the system. Behavior such as bookworming, sealing oneself up to study to the exclusion of all social interactive activity, is rewarded with better grades. With competition for entrance into medical school so fierce, the bookwormiest who have managed the top grades succeed in making it in and staying there. [p. 118]

Fifth, monopoly and autonomy create a special professional privilege which may separate professionals from dealing with the consequences of their decisions. The charter of autonomy includes the authority to define the terms of practice and "a legal, moral and intellectual mandate to determine for the individual and society at large what is healthy, moral, ethical, deviant, normal, or abnormal" (Reiff, 1974, p. 452). Thus, a system of logic and perception may be erected that organizes ethics and rationalization to protect professionals from the effects of their decisions. Those dependent on them suffer from their mistakes, ignorance, self-deception, and bias, since professionals define when a mistake has been made. In this way a situation is created in which feedback from experience is so limited that self-corrective action is less likely.

Sixth, by restricting entry to professions, licensing has created a situation in medicine where there are fewer practitioners per capita, and it is harder for people to find them and to afford to consult them. This artificial scarcity situation, according to sociologist Eliot Freidson (1970), encouraged physicians to practice on a "take it or leave it" basis, so that even more persons were denied service unless they were willing to conform to a physician's definition of the role of a good patient. Monopoly permits physicians to be unresponsive to market pressure because they, rather than their patients, determine demand (Carlson, 1970). One effect is observed by Gerstl and Jacobs (1976) as a shift in emphasis by professionals from control over quality to control of price. Another effect is to increase the distance between the professional and the client with the resulting difficulty of enlisting the patient as an ally in the treatment. Many patients are locked into a hierarchical and authoritarian relationship that devalues their contribution to health yet assigns guilt for their contribution to disease. The caring attitude necessary to meaningfully involve the patient in his or her own treatment, in spite of the existing knowledge about how important this is for quality outcomes, is less likely to occur under these circumstances.

In sum, it has been shown that licensing boards do not effectively determine initial competence of licensees, help to maintain their continued competence, effectively discipline errant practitioners, or properly address the needs of underserved populations. Instead, evidence has been presented showing that the licensing system has exacerbated the problems of maldistribution and underutilization of professionals, and supported a "licensing for life" system. Reviewing Roemer's (1970) conditions underlying high-quality service, shows that licensing systems generally do not impact on practice relevant to maintaining a safe and hygienic environment, developing an adequate supply of human resources, or enhancing access to resources. Material has been presented indicating that professions and professionals as they now operate tend to support patient-client dependency rather than foster an educated public. Licensing, then, does not make a positive contribution to these minimum, underlying requirements for good-quality care. The burgeoning self-help movement with its literature often written by professionals is officially ignored and privately derided by professionals. Given these findings, there does not seem to be any basis of support for the professional rhetoric that licensing protects the public by assuring minimal quality service. We are, in fact, tempted to speculate that it participates with other factors to ensure, instead, much less than competent service to a large number of Americans.

9

ALTERNATIVES TO PROFESSIONAL LICENSING

The import of this volume is to urge a change in policies concerning the credentialing of professionals, so that people may rely less on government and more on themselves. Many believe that the State has the obligation to protect people against quacks and incompetents. This has had the secondary effect of establishing the legitimacy of professions. Licensing has been effective in legitimating professions but does not effectively protect the public. Instead, people need help to rely more on their own ability to protect themselves against those who would harm and exploit them. People should be expected to assume a heightened degree of responsibility for themselves. The purpose of this chapter is to explore a variety of alternatives that would change the system of credentialing professions to one where public self-protection could become a reality on a large scale.

Change in the direction of less government and more self-reliance is not easy or immediately realizable. Difficult obstacles exist both in the standards of our entrenched guild-professions and in the dependency and mystification of the public. The present system has evolved over many generations; it will take time and effort to alter what we now encounter. Strong public support is necessary for organizations that pursue consumer interests and educate the public, literally from the cradle to the grave. Major developments are unlikely immediately, but advocacy agencies already exist (Shimberg, 1982) and information technology has placed more power in the hands of the consumer. Strategies can now be pursued that would increase the actual protection of the public and lead to the further development of a climate supportive of client self-protection.

A STRUCTURE FOR CHANGE

Referring to the special interests of bureaucrats who administer public service programs and the professionals who staff them, Freidson (1970) indicated that "Each perspective has its own legitimate interest that prevents it from adequate sensitivity to the perspectives of the patient" (p. 226). Clearly, there is a need to change these circumstances so that the public interest is primary. He offered several principles to consider in any effort to revise the means by which expert service is offered. While admitting that some type of bureaucratic system was necessary, Freidson argued for "indirect and parsimonious mechanisms open enough to allow a great deal of variety and flexibility in how they meet the standards they lay down" (p. 215). Crucial to this was the criterion that "the patient be in a position of sufficient independence to be able to exercise choice and have a voice in the organization, presentation, and substance of the care he gets" (p. 215). To accomplish these ends, attention must be paid to the social structure of the relationship between client and expert. This structure is presently formed by expert control of special knowledge which in turn is made possible through licensed monopoly and protected by self-regulated autonomy.

What consumers need but do not get is sufficient information, effective alternatives, accountability, reduced cost, and protection against those who would exploit their lack of knowledge. A more mutual relationship between professionals and their clients is essential in providing for such needs. Somers (1978) used the term *consumer sovereignty* to describe the need for the well-informed and responsible consumer. Altering the structure to achieve such ends requires change in the incentives that guide the behavior of both expert and client. Four types of incentives are needed: (1) incentives to encourage consumers to be self-determining and to use experts as advisers rather than as decision makers; (2) incentives for professionals to engage in public information and education programs; (3) incentives to enable valid assessment of competence, particularly in areas of service in which consumer ignorance and gullibility might lead to nonremediable consequences from inadequate service; and (4) incentives for professionals to provide data on the outcomes of intervention so accountability judgments may be made and the consumer information base enlarged. The alternatives suggested in the remainder of this chapter are steps toward providing these incentives. These alternatives are more indirect and parsimonious than Freidson's (1970) suggestion of creating dual systems to make service providers more competitive, Milgrom's (1978) statement that professional service should be regulated as are public utilities, or Havighurst's (1982) assertion that "the increased physician supply will contribute in due course to competition's emergence" (p. 94).

Many suggestions from within the professions about reforming the licensing system to increase its effectiveness involve "higher" standards, more control by already autonomous professionals, and consumer participation on regulatory boards. Competition has been an anathema to the professions but is suggested by critics and outsiders. Freidson (1970) (referring to the medical profession) insisted that "the circumstances of practice must be such as to require substantial competition of some kind among medical care institutions and practitioners for patients. Without such competition there is little likelihood that services will be responsive to the human needs of the clientele rather than only to those needs recognized by profession and administration" (p. 219). Pertschuk (1980), Commissioner and former chairman of the Federal Trade Commission, indicated that competition would act as an incentive for greater client self-determination and increased availability of information to the public.

> More and more consumers are discovering that professionals are not markedly different from other sellers who offer their services in trade. Nothing dissolves a mystique faster than seeing lawyers advertise inexpensive legal services just as used-car dealers advertise special deals. Making visible the commercial underpinnings of the professions is therapeutic. It fosters healthy skepticism, and teaches that, in this area as in all other commerce, a vigorous competition coupled with adequate consumer information ensures the optimum range of quality at the lowest possible price. [p. 346]

Recent Supreme Court decisions and activities of the Federal Trade Commission and the U.S. Department of Justice have promoted increased competition in the professions. In *Goldfarb* v. *Virginia State Bar* (1975) the argument that professions were exempt from antitrust laws was rejected. Overcast et al. (1982) pointed out that this led to investigations of professional practices restraining competition. The Department of Justice investigated architects, accountants, civil engineers, mechanical engineers, and physicians. The Federal Trade Commission investigated lawyers, accountants, real estate brokers, physicians, dentists, and veterinarians. Overcast et al. reasoned:

> Antitrust law is founded on the principle that competition is the touchstone for all commercial activity. Competitive markets tend to be more efficient and result in lower prices to consumers. Professional practice has many commercial aspects such as setting fees, establishing office procedures, purchasing equipment and supplies, billing clients, and obtaining referrals. . . . In antitrust litigation involving the activities of professional organizations, the courts are primarily concerned with answering the following question: Have the activities of the professional organization significantly impaired the ability of competitive market forces to determine (a) the price or fee for professional services, (b) who can enter the market, or (c) the degree of innovation within the profession? [p. 519]

Federal Trade Commission attempts to regulate anticompetitive business practices by professions recently bred a counterreaction. The House of Representatives passed but the Senate failed to approve a measure in December 1982 that would have restricted the FTC from jurisdiction over state-licensed professionals on consumer protection issues (Federal File, 1982).

Increased competition among service givers would counter the negative quality features of licensing that are associated with monopoly and autonomy. With information, clients could become increasingly self-determining and self-responsible. Service providers' interest in clients' needs would be enhanced, reducing arrogance and unresponsiveness. Efforts to educate clients would be undertaken, reducing dependency and mystification. Feedback from clients would be solicited, increasing awareness by service givers of the consequences of their decisions and of the outcome rather than just the process of interventions. Choice of alternative services would reduce reliance on narrow and less innovative services.

Competition would impact on professionalism as a defense of position, income, and property rights and focus professions more directly on their primary function of organizing knowledge. Ehrenreich (1978) indicated that a radical deprofessionalization is necessary if the health system is to be changed at all in the direction of including self-help and active patient modalities. Carlson (1976) saw the tie between regulation and professionalism. He justified deregulation by indicating that "many other reforms will founder unless professionalism is eroded" (p. 259).

Though competition theoretically only requires open entry to the field and sufficient information for consumers to make a choice, several factors make full implementation somewhat premature. The present dependency and mystification of the public and the high degree of inequality of information between practitioners and consumers, particularly regarding dangerous procedures, making choosing a complicated and risky process in some circumstances. So, as a result, the following proposals for changing the licensing system attempt to explore a middle ground between monopoly and unrestricted competition. Suggestions include: increasing the freedom of choice of practitioners by consumers, regulating dangerous procedures, regulating professional disclosure, using nongovernmental resources, educating both public and professionals for mutuality, and tying accountability to regulation. Though there are many proposals for the improvement of regulation we will cite here only those that assume that increased competition is necessary. Milton and Rose Friedman (1980) went to the extreme of unrestricted competition in proposing a simple and sweeping step, a constitutional amendment.

Few things have a greater effect on our lives than the occupations we follow. Widening freedom to choose in this area requires limiting the power of the states. The counterpart here in our Constitution is either the provision in its text which prohibits certain actions by states or the Fourteenth Amendment. One suggestion: *No State shall make or impose any law which shall abridge the right of any citizen of the United States to follow any occupation or profession of his choice.* [p. 305]

Kessell (1970) focused on health care as many do, since health care is such a problematic and expensive service. He argued that a mistake was made early in modern licensing history in specifying "how physicians were to be produced instead of specifying what the product should be . . ." (p. 281). His means of creating competition in the field of medicine would be to permit anyone to take the state licensing exams, without regard to how they acquired their knowledge and skill. He tied this more open access to a system of relicensure that would have all practitioners periodically required to take the same entry exam required of new candidates for licensure. He believed this would rid medicine of some of its worst practitioners. The California Board of Medical Quality Assurance (1982) included a redefinition of the scope of the practice of medicine, regulation of dangerous procedures, health practitioner registration, and professional disclosure.

INCREASE FREEDOM OF CHOICE

Removing the highly restrictive practice acts (which monopolize service areas) and substituting a less restrictive form of credentialing would be the means to facilitate entry of persons and occupations into markets monopolized by licensed occupations, thereby giving the public alternatives and increasing their arena for self-determination. Substituting *title* acts (which restrict the use only of the name of the profession) or *registration* acts (which only list providers) for *practice* acts (which restrict who can serve the public) and removing the legal and regulatory requirements which reserve third-party insurance and governmental payments for practitioners of licensed occupations would remove the most formidable of the existing barriers to freedom of choice.

Wolfson et al. (1980) indicated that in markets where there are deficiencies in information about services to be offered, a title act "provides consumers with information about the relative competence of alternative providers, [thus] smaller firms may be able to compete in quality with larger firms . . ." (p. 204). This in turn enhances the competitive vigor of the market.

Walter Gellhorn (1976) recommended a title act ". . . when a program of prior training or a demonstration of an objectively measureable degree of skill can be regarded as a genuine precondition of a person's claiming an occupational status" (p. 26). The title act permits the public to identify the trained "expert," but does not withdraw opportunity from those whose training was different from the orthodox or was accomplished via an apprenticeship. Registration, on the other hand, was recommended by Gellhorn for occupations that had difficulty in defining and measuring competence. Since registration is merely a listing of those who pursue an occupation, it has the advantage of identifying those persons without evaluating qualifications that cannot be clearly assessed. Substituting title and registration acts for practice acts would be a first step in reducing government involvement in the credentialing system. Substituting nongovernmental certification for these mechanisms would be a subsequent step in the directions of eliminating government involvement and obtaining a fuller freedom of choice. Any transition from a practice act to deregulation would probably require the sequence suggested because the public is so accustomed to regulation.

An immediate problem when less restrictive mechanisms are introduced is the danger of increased quackery. Havighurst (1982), proponent of deregulation in health care, thought the dangers of competition were overdrawn.

While such a choice-oriented policy lets people bear the bad consequences of their choices as well as enjoy the rewards (including savings from economizing), catastrophic mistakes would surely be rare in a system with sound incentives. . . . Because people—that is, consumers—can pool information, can join together voluntarily for the purpose of making informed choices, can gain allies and hire agents to help them in deciding, and can rely on reputable middlemen, their widely perceived ignorance and helplessness seem a false issue. . . . [p. 6]

There is danger of quackery even with licensing, as Carlson (1975) has said, because quackery "is unavoidable where money is made out of human suffering" (p. 224). This does not quiet the concerns about deregulation. Leonard Duhl (1977) said:

There are likely to be some people from what—oh how could we typify that—perhaps the fringe, who may in fact decide all of a sudden that they are practitioners in something called holistic or humanistic medicine, whom you characterize as maybe being ill-prepared in their very own discipline. What do we do about that? How do we in the pursuit of trying to find alternative forms of care that are more sensitive, more human, more personalized, how do we prevent consumers from being ripped off by charlatans in the process? [p. 8]

Table 9.1 examines these questions from Ullman's (1981) perspective. The remaining sections in this chapter attempt to answer these questions and quiet the anxiety they express. The suggestions and alternatives all assume a greater degree of competition and wider freedom of choice than now exists. As if in response, though, Barron (1966) reminded us that generally there are laws pertaining to truth in advertising, "fraud, violence, breach of contract, and other injurious conduct, together with procedures for redress of wrongs inflicted in the marketplace" (p. 661). The innovative California Board of Medical Quality Assurance (1982) pointed the way by providing for penalties for performing prohibited acts, unregistered practice, failure to observe disclosure requirements, causing harm, and false or misleading advertising. Further, the registration fee would cover an aggressive enforcement program.

TABLE 9.1 Analysis of Factors Influencing Dangerous Practice under Conditions of Free Consumer Choice

Factors That May Lead to an *Increase* in Ineffective or Dangerous Practice if Consumers Were Given Freedom of Choice	Questions That Put These Factors in the Broader Context of a Health Regulatory System
There may be more practitioners seeking to earn a living and thus there may be more practitioners seeking to make a "fast buck."	Will free market competition in health care raise or lower health care costs? Should income from a health practice be available only to medically educated practitioners?
New and untested practices may be developed that prove to be ineffective, dangerous, or may delay needed standard medical treatment.	Should unorthodox practices have to prove their efficacy when most medical procedures today have not? What beneficial or detrimental effects will result from delaying standard medical treatment?
The open marketplace may increase the amount of clinical experimentation on humans.	How much clinical experimentation in medicine takes place presently? What important innovations may result from this experimentation? What problems may result from this experimentation?
The increased involvement of consumers in their own health may create problems like: 1. Confusion over which practitioner has given the right diagnosis and best therapeutic plan 2. Increase in number of consumers worrying about what they can do for their health when sometimes little or nothing can be done 3. Lack of knowledge about how to obtain information related to their health 4. Lack of ability of consumers to judge some of the technical information in reference to their health	Will consumer involvement in their own health ultimately help or hinder their overall health? Is there value in obtaining a second opinion? Presently, are consumers not concerned enough with their health? Can an effective system be created to deal with this problem, and is it worth the expense? Are consumers smarter than professionals think? Can professionals make technical information understandable to consumers? Do consumers want to make their own decisions?

Source: Dana Ullman, "Regulate Freedom of Choice: An Alternative to Scope of Practice Licensure," paper presented at the American Public Health Association Conference, Detroit, November 1981. Reprinted with permission.

Table 9.1 (*continued*)

Factors That May Lead to a *Decrease* in Ineffective or Dangerous Practice if Consumers Were Given Freedom of Choice	Questions That Put These Factors in the Broader Context of a Health Regulatory System
The open marketplace may create competition in health care so that the less effective practitioners will not be able to maintain a practice.	Should health care primarily be considered a science, not a business? Is present health care already a business?
Students may be more encouraged to seek training in effective healing methods and only secondarily seek training that offers a degree or a license.	Is medical education the only way to train healers?
Fewer people may need potentially dangerous standard medical procecures because some of the unorthodox health practices will be therapeutically effective.	Which unorthodox health practices are effective? Which conditions or types of individuals tend to be helped more by unorthodox practices? How much can individuals trust their own experiences in determining if a practitioner has been helpful or harmful to them?
Establishing consumers as being primarily responsible for choosing their own health practitioner may generate greater numbers of people than ever becoming more actively involved in their own health care. More healthy life-styles may result.	Do consumers want to take responsibility for their own health? Are consumers capable of assuming primary responsibility for their own health?

REGULATE DANGEROUS PROCEDURES, NOT OCCUPATIONS

In the case where the present restrictions concerning who may practice an occupation are removed, there is a great deal of concern about the inappropriate use of potentially dangerous procedures. Licensing laws are thought to restrict the use of dangerous procedures to those professionals who meet the criteria set by state licensing boards for competency in the management of the procedure. The problem is how to remove unnecessary monopoly restrictions pertinent to the many nondangerous practices while at the same time protecting the public from dangerous incompetency. We have noted that the public in general is not presently nor in the foreseeable future likely to overcome its dependency on and mystification by professionals or remedy the inequality in information, all of which makes it relatively vulnerable to the use of dangerous procedures. It is all very well to say in areas where remedies are available as in the case of economic exploitation or denial of rights that it is appropriate for responsible consumers to take the consequences of poor decision making. But there is a reasonable limit to appropriate consumer responsibility. There is no remedy, for example, for botched surgery or mistaken evaluation of building stresses which lead to death, injury, disease, or disfigurement.

The procedures to be regulated should be those procedures that, when performed inadequately, have irremediable consequences. By regulating only those procedures with irremediable consequences, all legal and economic consequences would be excluded. Such losses may be redressed by other means. Interventions that lead to death, injury, disease, or disfigurement cannot be adequately remedied. Until the day arrives when consumers are able to make quality assessments about dangerous or shoddy services, such procedures should be regulated. Of course, much work needs to be done to determine which specific competencies fit these criteria, how they will be defined, and what procedures will be used, but it *is* within the realm of possibility to do so *if* we want to protect the public. It is more likely that competency would be validly and reliably assessed when it is more narrowly defined. Such evaluations should emphasize performance on criteria validated according to client outcomes.

In order that such regulation not be a way for presently licensed occupations to maintain their monopolies over particular procedures, all specialized competency evaluations should be open to anyone who has relevant training, regardless of occupation. The authority to prescribe restricted drugs, for example, might be given not only to physicians but also to pharmacists, psychologists, nurses, and others who could demonstrate competency on a valid and rigorous assessment. The pharmacists of the state of Washington have recently been given the right to prescribe drugs providing they work out an agreement with a provider (nurse-practitioner, physician's assistant, or physician) and submit the agreement to the pharmacy board for review. A report (APha, 1982) presented at the American Pharmaceutical Association compared pharmacists and physicians in prescribing drugs for mental health and ambulatory hypertensive patients. The pharmacists significantly outscored the physicians in overall quality of prescribing according to neutral judges using standard medical criteria.

A proposal before the California Board of Medical Quality Assurance (1982) would reserve the performance of dangerous activities to physicians or other specifically authorized licensed individuals. The dangerous activities included:

- Penetration of the tissues and surgery.
- Instrumentation beyond the vagina, mouth, and anus.
- Prescribing dangerous drugs.
- Use of ionizing radiation. [p. 4]

Later, the Board added "diagnosis of disease" (Proposal, 1982, p. 20).

REGULATE PROFESSIONAL DISCLOSURE

Information is at the center of any plan to enhance consumer self-protection. One problem to solve is that the result of the monopolization of knowledge by the licensed professions has been an inequality in the amount of information held by clients and professionals and in their influence over one another. To maintain power, professionals establish a social distance in which there is inequality in personal informational disclosure that develops a climate of mutual mistrust. Lopata (1976) reported that: "Particularly in personal service occupations, the client is expected to supply information about the self in order for the expert to convert generalized knowledge into relevant case application. The expert does not traditionally reveal any personal information about herself or himself" (p. 440). To do so weakens the authority of the professional. The authority rests on the sense of mystification created by the unequal information. If clients knew the professional as a person—"warts and all"—and if clients believed that they could know what professionals know, much of the structure responsible for dependency and for much of the placebo effect would disappear, the result being the equalizing of authority. However, the essential role of the professional—the organization and dissemination of knowledge—would remain. Reiff (1974) was convinced that "If the institutions of professionalism—its educational systems and organizations—were compelled to share their power with society, it would inevitably result in the democratization of knowledge and a new social contract between the professions and the society that supports them and the clients they serve" (p. 459). Gone too would be the strong supports for "the indifferent, dehumanized, self-perpetuating, entrepreneurial enterprise characteristic of professionalism today" (Reiff, 1974, p. 461). What would be gained would be the fuller participation of clients in their own problem solving, in the prevention of their problems, and in a maximizing of their potentials. To change the authority balance so it is more nearly equal, it is essential to permit more than just a small, already knowledgeable and assertive minority to become self-determining and self-responsible. Expecting consumers to protect themselves implies an informed, or at least informable, public. In this regard, Rogers (1973) quoted Richard Farson who believed, "The population which has the problem possesses the best resources for dealing with it" (p. 383). Consumers have the capacity and the responsibility to protect themselves. They have experience with the service and its consequences and the potential energy to do something about it. What they need is sufficient information to make sense of their experience and to overcome their mystifying dependence. It is clear that it is not knowledge but its control that is at the base of the inequality of authority. It follows, as Reiff (1974) has said: "If every professional were required to educate his clients and the public about what he is doing and why, the power of professionalism would be substantially weakened" (p. 460).

A second problem is posed if competition between service givers were to become a reality. In that case, it would be more likely that more information in the form of advertising would be directed at the public. According to a Federal Trade Commission (1979) report: ". . . an increase in the number of sellers in a market not only increases the number of potential sources of information; it also reduces the likelihood that sellers will be able to agree (either tacitly or through explicit collusion) to cut back on information dissemination" (p. 191). The converse is also true—increased information sources in most cases encourage competition by aiding the entry of new sellers into the market. This was the basis of FTC activity, which was directed at loosening self-imposed advertising restrictions in the professions. The FTC targeted physicians, dentists, accountants, veterinarians, and funeral directors. A Supreme Court decision (*Bates* v. *State Bar of Arizona*, 1977) and the voluntary removal of advertising prohibitions by private associations ultimately made FTC action unnecessary. The benefits noted by the FTC included reduced cost of consumer searching, increased competition, lower prices, increased access for new entrants, service to previously underserved groups in society, and an increase in alternative service providers. Specific drawbacks included a failure to affect other advertising-inhibiting restraints, an unsubstantiated concern that quality of service might be affected, and the need to police deceptive advertising.

Advertising is a fact of life in our highly mobile lives and in our anonymous communities. In effect, advertising replaces word of mouth and personal experience with products and services that existed in earlier times in communities where change was not a constant and communication channels actually reached most decision makers. The nineteenth century was identified as the height of the *caveat emptor* era in America, where "sellers apparently did not distinguish between giving consumers objective information and motivating them to buy. They seemed to recognize only two choices—provide truthful information or provide false information" (FTC, 1979, p. 148). In markets characterized by an oversupply, false and deceptive information became viable alternatives as sellers attempted to distinguish themselves from one another. False information increasingly became a target for regulation, but deceptive information (including such subjective claims as puffery, social-psychological claims, and nonverbal images) proved more difficult to control. The question of how to tailor restrictions on deceptive or unfair advertising so as not to stifle "truthful commercial speech" (FTC, 1979, p. 180) remains hard to answer.

The FTC has used "affirmative" disclosure of information as the "backbone of . . . [its] initiatives to enhance the quality and quantity of information available to consumers" (p. 276). Disclosure has been a remedy "for deception by omission or by misleading implications . . . [and] to correct unfairness generated by the imbalance in information availability between buyer and seller" (p. 276). Distinguished are "triggered" disclosures that are required when particular claims would be misleading if qualifying information were not given and "across-the-board" disclosures that are identified as applicable regardless of claims. The FTC report makes the following recommendations for enhancing the value of disclosures:

I. When consumers have no preexisting frame of reference for information, provide information about the desirable range of data and grading systems

II. Discontinue particular requirements when consumers develop the necessary frame of reference for evaluating information

III. Consider needs of target audiences by
   A. Using simple language
   B. Using disclosures that include brief and easily understood information along with more complex information in instances where a single disclosure does not meet the needs of all those involved

IV. Recognize multiple information channels
   A. Simplify broadcast disclosures
   B. Organize information at retail outlets
      1. For comparison of warranties
      2. For comparison of attributes
   C. Use labels especially when across-the-board disclosures are necessary

Regulating professional disclosure is a remedy for the inequality of authority and a means to restrain advertisers from false and deceptive claims. The following example (Gross, 1977) is drawn from specific experience with a professional statute for counselors, though it can be generalized for other professions. The first professional disclosure statute was written by Dan Elsass and Deborah Oughton of the State of Illinois House Minority staff, aided by Diane Reifler when she was training director at the OASIS Center for Human Potential in Chicago. Though it was not enacted into law, it does serve as an example of what is possible. Similar laws are pending in Michigan, Ohio, and Pennsylvania. It had the purpose of increasing consumer access to information relative to the quality of service available. It assumed that accurate information about the service offered by a practitioner was the consumer's best chance at getting what he or she wanted and needed and the best protection against harm and exploitation. It would give consumers information to aid in their evaluation of the competency of counselors and their compatibility with a particular client. In effect, it would restrict counselors, in this case, to doing what they say they were going to do.

The statute would provide a system of honest professional disclosure to prospective clients of those who designate themselves as counselors and the registration of this disclosure. It would not regulate who could or could not do counseling. Disclosure included name, business address and telephone number, philosophy of counseling, specifics of formal education, particulars of informal education and association memberships, and fee schedule.

The method by which the statute would be implemented included these provisions: (1) Disclosure was to be made to prospective clients before any counseling for which a fee may be charged. It was to be legible, on a printed form, and also posted conspicuously. (2) The fact that disclosure was required must be disclosed, including information about the particular department of state government that oversaw the procedure so that a complainant would know to whom a complaint was to be made. (3) A notarized form was to be filed annually or whenever a change in the statement was made. (4) Additional disclosure forms were necessary for supervisors and employers. (5) Complaints were to be made to the department of state government that had responsibility for investigation and public hearings. (6) Provision was made for privilege of counselor records during processing of complaints. (7) Judicial review of decisions was made possible. (8) The offense covered by the statute was the willful filing of false or incomplete information. (9) Punishment included the judgment of "misdemeanor" and the prohibition from practice.

There has been some interest in the counseling field in professional disclosure, though to date no law requiring professional disclosure has been implemented. Winborn (1977) used the concept of "honest labeling," but described a similar system of disclosure. Witmer (1978) did not think professional disclosure should stand alone but instead should be a part of a counselor licensing statute. Swanson (1979) showed how the disclosure concept could be used as an alternative to or a complement of a statement provided by a counselor in a community directory of counseling services. Gill (1982) offered some aid to counselors attempting to write such statements and gave some examples of statements appropriate for different settings. The California Board of Medical Quality Assurance (1982) proposal suggested professional disclosure as an alternative to licensure and tied it to a system of registration. Their proposal included the following:

Require unlicensed practitioners to register, file copies of disclosure statements, and document any claimed training.
  — Collect a registration fee to cover an aggressive enforcement program.
  — Specify parameters for use of titles, degrees, etc.

Registered practitioners would be required to give each patient full disclosure of
  — Training and education
  — Experience
  — What procedures the practitioner intends to offer or use
  — A disclaimer saying the State does not evaluate credentials, test competence, or in any way certify as to the practitioner's knowledge, competence, efficacy or safety.

Penalties: Stiff fines or other penalties for
  — Unregistered practice
  — Failure to observe disclosure requirements . . .
  — False or misleading advertising. [p. 6]

TIE ACCOUNTABILITY TO REGULATION

Recommended here has been a lessening of governmental involvement in the relationship between clients and professionals. Specifically, in substituting title and registration acts for practice acts, regulating dangerous procedures and requiring professional disclosure there would remain some governmental involvement in the client-practitioner relationship but procedures would be oriented toward competition, self-responsibility, and self-protection. Some continuing regulation is necessitated by the reality of client dependency and mystification and sustained by a continuing imbalance in the information available to clients and providers. It remains unclear, given the lack of experience with a highly responsible and self-protecting public, just how little regulation it is possible to live with and still deal with the legitimate vulnerability of clients to their more powerful "helpers." But it is clear that the regulation proposed is less onerous in the sense that it does not support provider monopoly and autonomy and does more to deliver protective circumstances to clients than does present reliance on licensing. Such regulation may then be considered an experiment to see how far a society can go in transferring responsibility to the public for its own protection and a transition from a noxious to a more ideal circumstance. Given the experimental nature of these proposals, it is necessary that feedback and evaluation be an essential part of the process. *Wherever there is regulation there should be accountability.*

Accountability is essentially the process of gathering information that permits the evaluation of the purposes, principles, procedures, relationships, results, and costs of an activity. Standards of accomplishment are developed against which the results of an activity may be explained, analyzed, or justified. The goal is to make action understood. Unfortunately, experience with accountability is not very encouraging nor is it clear how to accomplish it. Since the "state of the art" is realistically minimal given the lack of extensive experience, we catalogue some of the suggestions made to encourage accountability.

A recent review (Greer et al., 1978) of the accountability of public agency personnel emphasized the complexity of the problems and did not offer viable solutions. A review by Wolfson et al. (1980) of civil liability and standard setting as output regulators indicated these measures tended to fail for three reasons: (1) They required normally reluctant victims to initiate action, (2) they were very expensive in that they required a case-by-case assessment, and (3) they depended on an informed and assertive public for enforcement. Lieberman (1970) suggested state inspection programs and triple damages with return of attorney fees. Bucher and Stelling (1977) and Daniels (1973) suggested periodic and systematic performance reviews by panels which would include professionals from related disciplines and lay persons.

Bucher and Stelling (1977) encouraged physicians not to practice in isolation as increased visibility from group practice enhanced competence. They would also increase the public's awareness of its rights as clients, hold providers accountable for information given or not given to clients, and permit clients the right of access to any technical information professionals can provide, including availability of records for their own personal use as well as disguised records to be used for research and performance assessment. Annas (1976) insisted that PSRO data must be made available to the public, despite physician and hospital reluctance, if PSROs are to have any implication for public accountability. Mechanic (1979) suggested effective grievance procedures, ombudsmen, and increasing client pressure by informing clients of their rights and requiring meticulous and formal verification of consent.

Stewart and Cantor (1974) reported on client-oriented performance evaluations, which unfortunately did not appear to involve clients in the process. In such systems, measures of performance were updated periodically and criteria for performance measures were set jointly by professionals and managers in accord with client-oriented performance expectations. Operating the system was to be a joint activity between professionals and managers with the results to be fed into an information system. Lipsky (1978) despaired of bureaucratic methods of accountability and suggested increasing client control through service vouchers, program governance, and judicial relief. Maurizi (1980) examined the power of the client by studying consumer complaints. Perhaps facilitating consumer complaints will make a difference. A study of the Psychology Examining Committee for the California Department of Consumer Affairs (Summerfield, 1978) recommended that "A dignified sign be posted in every psychotherapist's office or place of consultation informing the patient that he has the right to file a complaint with the proper State agency, and that he may write or phone a toll free, 800 number. Such a sign would extract a cost in terms of an increased number of complaints received by the State agencies . . ." (pp. 110-11).

Brown (1978) discussed two aspects of the problem of accountability. He noted that consumers of health care were observers of the system rather than participants because their feedback was not incorporated in the service provided. He also noted the disinclinations of physicians to receive criticism. They tended to question the criteria used to make the judgment rather than their own performance. The system was not prepared to receive feedback nor was the consumer prepared to give it. The validity and reliability of the measures left much to be desired as did the disinterest of professionals. Perhaps the central notion is the acceptance of the importance of the client role. Stewart and Cantor (1974) paraphrase Howard Vollmer: ". . . occupational groups must be evaluated eventually by the clientele because the clientele provide the basic rationale for the existence of the occupation. Evaluation of performance by the client can lead to less control by the occupation and more control for the client, thus less autonomy for the worker . . ." (p. 349).

In the instance that client reaction was the central unit in an accountability system, Bernstein and Lecomte (1981) suggested a client self-report evaluation form sent to a regulating agency. "Confidentiality and restricted access to raw data would be strictly enforced, and periodic summaries of client evaluations would be available to the therapist and potential clients" (p. 206). They also suggested that therapists report client outcomes in a system conducted jointly with clients to provide some balance for the consumer data. The relationship between accountability, regulation, and an enlightened, responsible, and self-protecting public is the extent to which data exist and are made evident to show that the regulation is achieving the ends desired. It is hard to see how client data, whether self-report, unobtrusive measures, or behavioral observation, can be anything but central to the enterprise.

NONGOVERNMENTAL RESOURCES

Opening up access to service delivery by competing providers would stimulate several nongovernmental initiatives. Professional associations would be spurred to develop their own certifying agencies to inform the public about the competence of their members. In the competition among professional groups, it would become advantageous for certification to rely on measures predictive of quality performance lest the professions lose out in striving for public acceptance and credibility. There would be incentives for professional groups to educate the public, if only to assure respect for the expertise of their particular professional groups. Consumer groups would encourage client self-responsibility by publicizing the rights of patients and by advocating the use of informed consent agreements and contracts. The public is likely to desire more information and education once they realize what has always been true, that there is no one "out there" protecting them.

Voluntary Certification

Voluntary certification is national in character and certifying agencies are free to stress standards that genuinely emphasize competence. Such a system does not prevent uncertified persons from being hired, though some employers may stipulate certification as a qualification. The major weakness of such a system is the absence of any standards regarding the quality of the credentials issued. Shimberg (1980) said that: "Any group wishing to establish its own certification agency is free to do so. . . . There is no way of knowing how much credence to place in a certification credential without also knowing how trustworthy the certification agency is and what standards it applies in awarding its credentials" (p. 21).

Recognizing this potentiality and wishing to develop an alternative to state licensing, a U.S. Department of Health, Education, and Welfare committee (Cohen, 1976) recommended the establishment of a national certification council to approve certification organizations and the development of national standards for the credentialing of health organizations. The National Commission for Health Certifying Agencies (NCHCA) was chartered in 1977 to establish such order and credibility in health profession credentialing. It functions as an accrediting agency by evaluating certifying bodies rather than actually certifying anyone itself. The Commission is most sensitive to the issue of being co-opted by the professional organizations.

In a period of increasing doubt about the capacity and vigor of health professions in regulating themselves, the viability of certification depends on great strides in improving techniques of certification to increase job-relatedness, better assure entry-level and continuing competence and enhance the accountability to the public of mechanisms of professionalization. [Falk et al., 1980, p. 99]

The Commission goes about this duty by setting standards for membership. The criteria for the standards include service by the standard to the public interest, universality of application to all professions, and the practical attainability of standards. The standards touch on agency structure, examination process, dissemination of information to the public, and efforts by the agency to update procedures in light of new knowledge about occupational credentialing. The agencies must be nongovernmental and nonprofit; be administratively independent from professional associations; have boards broadly representative of the public, the profession, and employees; have access to authoritative consultation in examination construction; and be financially secure. Discriminating practices that would exclude persons on the basis of age, sex, race, religion, national origin, disability, or marital status are forbidden. Agencies are also required to establish alternate pathways as an option for educational requirements. To date, twenty certifying agencies are members of the Commission.

Shimberg (1980) was hopeful about the growth of credentialing agencies: "Insurance companies and other third party payors . . . [want] assurance that those providing services are, in fact, qualified to render them" (p. 24). He also expected that certification might fill the gap at such time when state licensing is no longer considered sufficient for qualification as a provider under federally funded programs. This latter point is a good sign for the Commission and for certification generally. If the Commission's stringent requirements were to become widely accepted, there would be widespread impact on credentialing practice. Nathan Hersey was quoted (Licensure Efforts, 1982) as saying that the most dramatic issue today for health groups was establishing qualifications for direct reimbursement.

Performance-Based Evaluation of Competence

Professional associations will regain credibility to the extent their competency measures predict quality performance. Williamson's (1976) review of research on the relation of certification to actual clinical performance concluded: "certification results, whether measured by professional undergraduate grades or medical specialty certification examinations, seem to have very little relationship to quality of subsequent professional performance" (p. 25). In a system where the public has options, there is a need to develop ways to make it possible for potential providers to demonstrate competence without regard to how it is acquired. Competence and education are not equivalent. Strong resistance to change should be expected from the professions. Pottinger (1980b) detailed the politics of change using the example of the health professions. Marketability and status of the health professionals are tied to academic credentials, licenses, and tests of knowledge retention. The tests have been biased in favor of those who are formally educated, emphasizing as they do questions based on knowledge relevant to curriculum rather than to job performance. Professions naturally resist transferring their wealth by preventing the competent but "uneducated" from diluting their status. By so doing, they maintain their market value in the health care delivery system. Support for alternative career entry paths, for example through apprenticeship training and proficiency testing, hold the promise of circumventing "the very trappings that give the professions their marketability" (p. 14). Though the federal government has led in the effort to support those competent workers lacking formal education, the politics are such that accreditation and reimbursement policies that identify acceptable practitioners must also change so that the incentive system rewards competence rather than merely credentials. It is hard to say at this point whether sharply rising costs in the health care sector will offer sufficient basis to overcome the entrenched resistance to change where professional monopolies are presently sustained not by demonstrable benefits to the public but by a reimbursement system. The National Commission's standard requiring alternative paths is an encouraging sign, presently.

The neglect of competency assessment by the professions has not been for lack of theory and research but rather for lack of will. The decision about what to measure and what not to measure demonstrates particular values and becomes an instrument of social policy. If social instrumentalities are to serve people, measurement of competency should attend to variables that inform the public about the likely effectiveness of a given service. If competency measurement is to perform this function, public policy requires a definition of competency that goes beyond knowledge retention and its regurgitation. Rather, it should integrate an understanding of the characteristics of the person performing a service with an understanding of the situations in which the person is to perform that service.

Though competency-based assessment is a reality in diverse areas of human services and the technology is available, funding barriers and a system that rewards educational credentials stand in the way of further development. Methods (described in chapter 7), including assessment center, behavioral events, and job analyses based on the personal competencies that cause superior performance appear promising.

Contracts

Green (1978) discussed the contract as a means of allocating responsibility between client and provider and as the framework for the building of personal relationships. Contracts clarify understandings and expectations, thereby shaping the relationship. It is in this sense that contracting has implication for supporting client self-responsibility and self-protection. Contracts that inform clients and buld suitable expectations about self-responsibility can enhance client responsibility. Contracts ordinarily include a definition of each party's responsibility, a statement of some common purpose, and an indicaton of the length of time the contract is to be in effect. Contracts should also stipulate methods of payment, clarify questions of client access to professional records, and indicate how and when they will be terminated, modified, or renewed. Green (1982) urged participants to avoid disclaimers or waivers of liability as these are usually ignored by the courts as being against public policy or may become part of an argument about unlawful intent. Green (1978) takes pains to point out that the formal contract is not the only contract possible.

A paper titled "Contract" is simply evidence of . . . an agreement. Other evidence may include the behavior of the parties, notes and records, material used in the performance of the agreement, and testimony of witnesses to conversation between the parties. In other words, the contract is the conceptualization of the relationship. It is the responsibility of the parties to define their relationship in a way which clarifies their mutual expectations. [pp. 392-93]

Green (1978, 1982) and Morrison (1979) indicated that contracts may be used to substitute for informal consent agreements, to provide a means to avoid malpractice charges, and to serve as the basis for providing alternative health care not in conflict with medical practice laws. Green (1982) cautioned that their validity in these matters had not had a binding court test. In the case of a challenge to contracts he indicated that the most likely principle to be used in deciding the issues will be reasonableness, given the inequality of information client and provider bring to the relationship. Information disclosure by the provider, here too, is crucial to any evaluation of reasonableness. Green (1982) showed that good agreements, information, and encouragement of self-responsibility all go hand in hand.

If the making of agreements is undertaken as a clarification of the planning process and its purpose to further the working relationship, this will increase the likelihood of achieving expectations. The making of agreements will minimize the risk of misunderstandings which can lead to failure in the relationship and disputes over responsibility. The thoughtfulness with which agreements are made is fundamental in determining whether the agreement will withstand a challenge to its validity. [p. 13]

He suggested that beginning agreements should be as simple as possible. Discussing the agreement uncovers expectations that may lead to disappointment had they remained implicit. Since experience with contracts is limited, rather than writing them out Green suggested living with verbal agreements —testing all the while how they fit the practice and the clients. Not insisting on a written contract to begin with also permits individual differences in agreements pertinent to the different needs of both providers and clients in differing circumstances.

Contracting enhances alternative ways for professionals to serve clients by stimulating professionals to share information and stimulating clients to make decisions. Contracts also may provide the basis for encouraging the entry of new professionals into the marketplace, furthering competition by creating a system for alternative approaches to be legally offered even where restrictive licensing laws are in effect. Finally, by stimulating disclosure, contracting carries the seeds of a strategy of altering authoritative-dependency practitioner-client relationships.

CONTINUING EDUCATION FOR MUTUALITY

Most people believe that professional licensing protects them. It is important to understand, if constructive alternatives are to be developed, that the present system meets the perceived needs of many of the public and most of the professionals. The true needs of the public also must be clear. We have seen that the public tolerates its present position of dependency because access to information concerning self-protection and self-determination is difficult to obtain and because assertiveness in this realm raises the threatening possibility of abandonment by professionals. The threat is posed that a professional's expertise may be the key to personal survival. Professionals are seen to bring order to an otherwise chaotic and dangerous world. Although this attitude accounts for consumer resistance to change and partly explains the basis for a portion of the power that remains entrenched with professionals, it also has encouraging aspects, suggesting that increasing public knowledge and self-determination is the key to reform.

The dominant-submissive power equation could be upset. Alford (1975) suggested the need for a changing consciousness among consumers about the adequacy of present protective measures to lay the groundwork for a challenge to entrenched interests. Carlson (1975) saw a new consciousness developing that will make it possible for people to assume more responsibility in caring for their own needs. Theobold (1972) saw this coming about in the societal shifts to a type of thinking that emphasized feedback about the consequences of behavior and deemphasized goal-directed behavior. Defined as nonlinear, this thinking has been evidenced in the growing concern about environmental issues. Lieberman (1970) did not believe a vital society could result from a "social system which defeats the incentives for self-help" (p. 275). Mechanic (1976), citing the abortion issue, observed that "people in modern societies are seeking greater autonomy over decisions affecting their own lives" (p. 14). Focusing on the licensure issue specifically, Engel and Hall (1973) indicated that change in professional work patterns was brewing. They cited the guild system—the precursor of modern professionalism—as having broken down under conditions similar to those present today when faced with demands of sharply increasing knowledge and technology, public desires for more and newer products, the need to increase outputs and lower costs, and pressure from other occupations to enter the system.

Though substantial change appears unlikely at this time—given the entrenched power of experts, the tenacity with which experts withhold knowledge, and the increasing complexity of that knowledge—there is reason to believe that the direction for change is through public awareness. Mechanic (1976) indicated that the process had already begun, referring to physicians' special prerogatives which have

been eroded by public criticism of the profession, by increased sophistication of consumers, by the growing organization and militancy of other health professions that are increasingly challenging the special position of the physician, and by changing the character of medical care itself which is undermining the very special ties between patients and individual physicians. [p. 175]

Roth (1975) cited women's health groups as a model for change in decision-making power.

Members of such women's groups provide much of their own health care without the intervention of "experts," make decisions on when the help of specially-trained experts will be useful, take part in selecting which technicians or consultants will be utilized, and specify the conditions and the manner in which this service will be provided. [p. 6]

He added, "If such an approach could be used by all of us with respect to our own health, not only would much of the decision-making power be in the hands of the consumer instead of the professional expert, but certified professionals would be far less often needed and the size and complexity of health service occupations could be considerably reduced" (p. 6).

The public has two interdependent disadvantages in relationships with professionals. Remedying the primary disadvantage, that of relative ignorance, requires remedying the second, the professional monopoly, by enhancing freedom of choice. However, the politics of gaining freedom of choice require, in turn, a public aware of its power. The mystification of the public about its power in the relationship with professionals is crucial to maintaining the status quo. False hope on the part of consumers that professionals will protect them was, according to Carlson (1975), the "major obstacle to reform" (p. 219). The entire superstructure of professional dominance relies on the consumer's belief that the expert knows best. Needed, according to Lieberman (1970), were "the tools and means by which we can comprehend the claims of experts and puncture their pretensions" (p. 262). Increasing consumer knowledge so that more mutual relationships can develop is the first step in a strategy emphasizing self-protection by the public itself.

The need for mutuality in relationships between professionals and clients is nowhere more evident than in the health care arena. In their relationships with professionals, patients are locked into hierarchical, authoritarian relationships that devalue their individual contributions to health and simultaneously assign guilt for their contribution to disease. At present, an approach is supported that encourages people to look beyond themselves (to a physician, to a pill) to learn what is good for them, which, in turn, prevents them from making meaningful contributions to their own health.

Less restrictive regulation and increased information would place the client in the position of having more independent and knowledgeable individual choice. With such a structure, it might then be likely to see the role of the professional change from decision maker to adviser. Mechanic (1976) indicated that information has already changed some physician-patient relationships:

the sophisticated consumer is increasingly straining the traditional doctor-patient relationship and challenging the authority of the physician in a fashion that many physicians find uncomfortable. As the momentum for consumer input grows, or support for encouraging informed and articulate patients develops, and as the public increasingly becomes more sophisticated about medical science and medical practice, the character of traditional physician-patient relationships will change significantly. [pp. 18-19]

Developing the ability of the public to enter into relationships with professionals in mutuality does not mean that the public would supplant professionals, but rather that the authority of professionals would be reestablished at a level consonant with the value of information and treatments they provide. For professionals, this means they will need to learn to respect the opinions of other, hitherto suppressed, experts and the judgment of clients to know what is best for themselves. Mutuality is defined as a sharing of decision-making authority and where status and prestige are unaffected by the roles one undertakes or their position in a hierarchy.

Mutually characterizes a relationship in which individuals are able to contribute their differing talents, these differing talents are respected, and each party to the relationship learns something from the other. In all of this, there would be a major role for continuing education, not only of professionals, but also for the public.

The ways to provide consumer education are, of course, varied and, given the extent of the job to be done, open to more creative and effective modalities. Newman and Kramer (1979) discussed the advantage of training teachers who are in touch with the needs of indigenous communities as opposed to direct consumer education by experts. Their project provided information and curriculum materials to aid consumers on how to avoid frauds in purchasing goods and services and how to complain effectively. Ng, et al. (1978) proposed the health promotion organization (HPO) as an educational alternative to the health maintenance organization. HPOs would create incentives and educate the public to value healthy life-styles and to take responsibility for their own health. HPOs would work with individuals and would coordinate relationships among government, business, labor, and the health care system. The HPO could become a part of existing health care facilities and be the vehicle to incorporate nonmedical expertise and self-help approaches into the traditional system.

Self-help is an important force for consumer education as well as an alternative to professional service. The self-help movement has been characterized by two educational goals important to the public in their relationships with professionals. The first is the information essential to self-care, particularly in those areas where professional monopolization of knowledge has appeared to be biased or limited, as in the case of women's medical issues (for example, women's anatomy, sexuality, birth control, and so on). The second is the training of consumers in how to select a service provider, how to know when one is needed, how to evaluate the service performed, and how to go about redressing grievances about the quality and the cost of service. Andrews and Levin (1979) discuss the self-care movement evident in both the extensive literature available on any paperback-book rack and the explicit instruction available in a wide variety of educational and service settings. They note two models. One trains the patient to be a member of the medical team emphasizing promotion of health, prevention of disease, health monitoring, control of medication, and so on. A second model trains patients to be as autonomous as their time, effort, and interest allow. There is probably a desirable limit to patient involvement, however. John Ehrenreich (1978) argued that some professional technologies were clearly useful but at the same time inappropriate for untrained people to use. He called for a redirecting of dependency in a society where freedom of choice existed. "What we have to develop is a medical system which acknowledges our need for for autonomous control over our bodies and which accepts our need for dependency; which enhances autonomy but, when we do feel the necessity to give up and be dependent, can deal with that need in a dignified and nurturing way" (pp. 27-28).

In relationships characterized by mutuality, professionals are respectfully attentive to clients, act as advisers and educators, and acknowledge their limitations. To achieve such changes in role, professional preservice and continuing education will need to change. Preparing a professional for mutuality in client-professional relationships and for taking on an advisory role in decision making is very different indeed from current training which emphasizes autonomy and distance from clients in relationships and the decision-maker roles. Professional educational institutions will need to change their emphasis in selection from those who are excellent "thing"-oriented regurgitators of scientific knowledge to those who are excellent people-oriented appliers of knowledge. The emphasis in preservice and continuing education will need to shift to caring and the uses of knowledge.

Lenrow (1978) supported the concept of mutuality but suggested a restructuring of how service is offered in the helping relationship. There was a need

to make oneself clearly accountable to the clients for the effects of exercising one's skills. This involves the development of a working relationship in which the clients have the power to define the problem in their own terms, to specify values that must be included in a solution, to use the helper to generate most alternatives from which they can choose, to select other helpers in addition to or instead of a particular professional, and to decide when they no longer need help. [pp. 284-85]

Lenrow did not entirely trust the professional helper to be objective enough. He believed it necessary to include a partner for the professional who would be responsible for a dialogue that could take place in the client's presence. The dialogue would focus on the limitations of the professional as they may affect the client. Without such a structure, individual professionals would "contribute to confusion, role-conflict, and negative side-effects in their well-intentioned efforts" (p. 285).

Marieskind's (1976) study, reported in table 9.2, of the knowledge held by clients under three types of clinic conditions is suggestive of the types of outcomes that might be expected with more mutuality in the exchange of knowledge: a physician-staffed traditional clinic; a clinic staffed by physician-trained paramedics; and a feminist self-help-facility.

Though Marieskind did not report statistical significance levels for the differences between the groups or control for selective factors, if knowledge retained is any measure of the conditions under which it is disseminated, patient autonomy and provider advice appear to be more effective than professional autonomy and patient dependency.

We have noted the comments of observers that the increasing sophistication of consumers is currently putting a strain on some professional-client relationships. The self-help, self-care, and consumer movements are indica-

TABLE 9.2 Correct Scores of Knowledge Measurements of Women in
Three Types of Medical Facilities (Percentages)

Test	Traditional	Paramedic	Self-Help	All Facilities
Anatomy identification (clitoris, uterus, vagina, os, Fallopian tube, urethra, ovary, labia, cervix, hymen)	46.2	54.6	72.2	57.7
Definition of gynecological procedures (Breast exam, Pap smear, speculum, pelvic exam, D&C, biopsy)	82.0	85.6	98.0	88.6
Knowledge of appropriate frequency of performing procedures	60.0	67.6	73.2	67.0
Contraceptive Contraindications (Pill, IUD, diaphragm, foam, condom)	22.0	39.2	39.2	33.4

Source: H. I. Marieskind, "Helping Oneself to Health," *Social Policy,* 1976, 7(2), 65. *Social Policy* is published by Social Policy Corporation, New York, New York 10036. Copyright 1976 by Social Policy Corporation.

tions of a growing trend in American society to call an end to the distance maintained by professionals from their clients, which has resulted in an exceedingly costly and ineffective system of professional dominance in provider services. There is no "going back," as these changes have been generated by mass education and communications. They give the lie to the necessity for professional monopolization of knowledge. The bottom line, of course, in any educational strategy is not whether information has been disseminated but whether, and the extent to which, learners are stimulated to do something about what they have learned. It seems more likely that such action would occur as a result of more freedom of choice of professional providers and more explicit attempts to train people to participate and be more sophisticated about the choice of a professional when one is needed, whether the need is for physician, attorney, architect, or accountant. For the future, it is likely that computers and communication technology together will transform information dissemination and, in turn, the relationships between providers and consumers in ways that may only be guessed today. The writers of the proposal to revise the California Medical Practice Act (Board, 1982) envisioned changes in health care as striking as the change in emphasis from infectious disease management to the care of chronic and degenerative disease that has occurred over the past several decades. They argued that the future would judge what we now consider central to health care to be as "antiquated as leeches. It does not seem outlandish to envision home computer programs which could diagnose most common conditions, provide self-care regimens and warn people when it is appropriate to consult a physician" (p. 26).

The fact that the issue of licensing the health professions has erupted again in the last decade after lying dormant for a century is an expression of the changes in the social and economic structures of the society. The relationship between consumers and professionals must change in response to changes in the central function of that relationship—the exchange of information. It is clear that licensing—the legal structure defining that relationship in the health professions—is rigid and antiquated and not up to accommodating the necessary change. New structures similar to those suggested in this chapter are necessary to permit greater flexibility in consumer-provider relationships and to transform the ineffective and inefficient system of "protection of the public" into viable strategies for consumer self-protection. In an infomation-based society, it is possible.

BIBLIOGRAPHY

Alford, R. R. *Health care politics*. Chicago: University of Chicago Press, 1975.

American Psychological Association, Division of Industrial-Organizational Psychology. *Principles for the validation and use of personnel selection procedures*. 2d ed. Berkeley, Calif.: Author, 1980.

Annas, G. J. Public access to health care informaton. In R. H. Egdahl and P. M. Gertman, eds., *Quality assurance in health care*. Germantown, Md.: Aspen System Corporation, 1976.

Andrews, L. B., and Levin, L. S. A review of the medical practice acts in light of developments in self care. *Social Policy*, 1979, *9*(4), 44-49.

APha presents evidence. *Professional Regulation News*, 1982, *1*(10), 4.

Arizona senator, in reform effort, asks end to continuing education requirements. *ProForum*, 1980, *2*(9), 7.

Augustine, A. More on gray areas. *ProForum*, 1979, *2*(2), 8.

Barber, B. Some problems in the sociology of the professions. In K. S. Lynn, ed., *The professions in America*. Boston: Houghton-Mifflin, 1965.

Barron, J. F. Business and professional licensing—California, a representative example. *Stanford Law Review*, 1966 *18*, 640-55.

Bates v. State Bar of Arizona, 433 U.S. 350 (1977).

Begun, J. W. *Professionalism and the public interest: Price and quality in optometry*. Cambridge, Mass.: MIT Press, 1980.

Benham, L. The effect of advertising on the price of eyeglasses. *Journal of Law and Economics*, 1972, *15*(2), 337-52.

_____. The demand for occupational licensure. In S. Rottenberg, ed., *Occupational licensure and regulation*. Washington, D.C.: American Enterprise Institute, 1980.

Benham, L., and Benham, A. Regulating through the professions: A perspective on information control. *Journal of Law and Economics*, 1975, *18*(2), 421-48.

Benham, L.; Maurizi, A.; and Reder, M. W. Migration, location and remuneration of medical personnel: Physicians and dentists. *The Review of Economics and Statistics*, 1968, *50*(3), 332-47.

Bernstein, B., and Lecomte, C. Licensure in psychology: Alternative directions. *Professional Psychology*, 1981, *12*(2), 200-8.

Bernstein, M. *Regulating business by independent commission*. Princeton, N.J.: Princeton University Press, 1955.

Blair, R. D., and Kaserman, D. L. Preservation of quality and sanctions within the professions. In R. D. Blair and D. L. Kaserman, eds., *Regulating the professions*. Lexington, Mass.: D. C. Heath, 1980.

Bledstein, B. J. *The culture of professionalism*. New York: Norton, 1976.

Bloom, S. W., and Wilson, R. N. Patient-practitioner relationships. In H. E. Freeman, S. Levine, and L. G. Reeder, eds., *Handbook of medical sociology*. Englewood Cliffs, N.J.: Prentice-Hall, 1972.

Board of Medical Quality Assurance. *2052 study: The legal definition of the practice of medicine*. State of California Department of Consumer Affairs, 1982.

Bond, R. S.; Kwoka, T. E., Jr.; Phelan, J. J.; and Whitten, I. T. *Effects of restrictions on advertising and commercial practice in the professions: The case of optometry*. Washington, D.C.: U.S. Government Printing Office, 1980.

Bosk, C. L. Defining and regulating the professions: The Quebec experience. *Annals of Internal Medicine*, 1977, *87*(5), 628-29.

Boston Women's Health Book Collective. *Our bodies, ourselves*. New York: Simon and Schuster, 1973.

Boyatzis, R. E. Competence at work. In A. J. Stewart, ed., *Motivation and society*. San Francisco: Jossey-Bass, 1982.

Bray, D. W. The assessment center and the study of lives. *American Psychologist*, 1982, *37*(2), 180-89.

Bray, D. W.; Campbell, R. J.; and Grant, D. L. *Formative years in business: A long-term AT&T study of managerial lives*. New York: Wiley, 1974.

Breyer, S. Different modes of classical regulation and their problems. In R. S. Gordon, ed., *Issues in health care regulation*. New York: McGraw-Hill, 1980.

Brown, J.H.U. *The politics of health care*. Cambridge, Mass.: Ballinger, 1978.

Brown, W. F., and Cassady, R., Jr. Guild pricing in the service trades. *Quarterly Journal of Economics*, 1947, *61*(2), 311-38.

Bucher, R., and Stelling, J. G. *Becoming professional*. Beverly Hills, Calif.: Sage Publications, 1977.

Carlson, R. J. Health manpower licensing and emerging institutional responsibility for the quality of care. *Law and Contemporary Problems*, 1970, *35*, 849-78.

_____. *The end of medicine*. New York: Wiley, 1975.

_____. Alternative legislative strategies for licensure: Licensure and health. In R. H. Egdahl and P. M. Gertman, eds., *Quality assurance in health care*. Germantown, Md.: Aspen Systems Corporation, 1976.

Carman, H. G. The historical development of licensing for the professions. *The Educational Record*, 1958, *39*, 268-78.

Carroll, S. L., and Gaston, R. J. *Occupational licensing: Final report*. National Science Foundation Grant Apr. 75-16792, October 31, 1977.

_____. Barriers to occupational licensing of veterinarians and the incidence of animal disease. *Agricultural Economic Review*, 1978, 37-39.

_____. State occupational licensing provisions and quality of service: The real estate business. *Research in Law and Economics*, 1979a, *1*, 1-14.

_____. Examination pass rates as entry restrictions into licensed occupations. *Midsouth Journal of Economics*, 1979b, *3*, 1-5.

_____. A note on the quality of legal services: Peer review and disciplinary service. *Research in Law and Economics*, 1981a, *3*, 251-60.

_____. Occupational restrictions and the quality of service received. *Southern Economic Journal*, 1981b, *47*(4), 959-76.

Challes, D. Holistic medicine education. *Holistic Health Review*, 1979, *3*(2), 118.

Chase, R. A., and Burg, F. D. Reexamination/recertification. *Archives of Surgery*, 1977, *112*(1), 22.

Christoffel, T. *Health and the law: A handbook for health professionals*. New York: Free Press, 1982.

Clarkson, K., and Muris, T. The Federal Trade Commission and occupational regulation. In S. Rottenberg, ed., *Occupational licensure and regulation*. Washington, D.C.: American Enterprise Institute, 1980.

Clemons, S.; Blaylock, K.; and McGowan, A. M. *Arkansas state regulation vs. the public interest*. Little Rock: Arkansas Consumer Research, 1981.

Cohen, H. S. Professional licensure, organizational behavior, and the public interest. *Milbank Memorial Fund Quarterly*, 1973, *51*(1), 73-83.

_____. Regulatory politics and American medicine. *American Behavioral Scientist*, 1975, *19*(1), 122-36.

_____. *A proposal for credentialing health manpower*. Rockville, Md.: Health Resources Administration, Public Health Service, U.S. Department of Health, Education, and Welfare, 1976.

Cohen, H. S., and Miike, L. H. Toward a more responsive system of professional licensure. *International Journal of Health Services*, 1974, *4*(2), 265-72.

Cohen, R. J. *Malpractice, A guide for mental health professionals*. New York: Free Press, 1979.

Collins, R. *The credential society: An historical sociology of education and stratification*. New York: Academic Press, 1979.

Consumer's resource handbook. Washington, D.C.: U.S. Government Printing Office, 1982.

Continuing education does not lead to continuing competency. *ProForum*, 1979, *2*(4), 5.

Cottingham, H. F. School counselors face the question of licensing. *School Counselor*, 1975, *22*, 255-58.

Council of State Governments. *Occupational licensing regulation in the states*. Chicago: Author, 1952.

Cummings, N. A. Turning bread into stones—Our modern antimiracle. *American Psychologist*, 1979, *34*(12), 1119-29.

Daniels, A. K. How free should professionals be? In E. Freidson, ed., *The professions and their prospects*. Beverly Hills, Calif.: Sage Publications, 1973.

Danish, S. J., and Smyer, M. A. Unintended consequences of requiring a license to help. *American Psychologist*, 1981, *36*(1), 13-21.

Dent v. State of West Virginia, 129 U.S. 114 (1889).

Department of Health, Education, and Welfare. *Report on licensure and related health personnel credentialing*. Washington, D.C.: U.S. Government Printing Office, 1971.

_____. *Health resources statistics: Health manpower and health facilities, 1974*. Washington, D.C.: U.S. Government Printing Office, 1974.

_____. *A proposal for credentialing health manpower*. Washington, D.C.: U.S. Government Printing Office, 1976.

_____. *Health resources statistics: Health manpower and health troubles, 1976-1977 Edition*. Washington, D.C.: U.S. Government Printing Office, 1979.

Derbyshire, R. C. *Medical licensing and discipline in the United States.* Baltimore: Johns Hopkins Press, 1969.

_____. Medical ethics and discipline. *American Medical Association Journal,* 1974, *228,* 59-63.

_____. Physician competence. What is the problem? What are the answers? *New York State Journal of Medicine,* 1979, *79*(7), 1028-31.

Dolan, A. K. Occupational licensure and obstruction of change in the health care delivery system: Some recent developments. In R. D. Blair and S. Rubin, eds., *Regulating the professions.* Lexington, Mass.: D. C. Heath, 1980.

_____. The law and the maverick health practitioner. *St. Louis University Law Journal,* 1982, *26*(3), 627-78.

Donabedian, A. Models for organizing the delivery of personal health services and criteria for evaluating them. *Milbank Memorial Fund Quarterly,* 1972, *50*(part 2), 120-22.

Donnison, J. *Midwives and medical men. A history of inter-professional rivalries and women's rights.* London: Heinemann, 1977.

Dörken, H. Avenues to legislative success. *American Psychologist,* 1977, *32,* 738-45.

Duhl, L. Testimony before California Assembly Health Committee. *Humanistic Medicine and Holistic Health Care.* Sacramento: State of California, 1977.

Efforts expand to check professional misconduct. *ProForum,* 1978, *1*(5), 3.

Ehrenreich, J., ed. *The cultural crisis of modern medicine.* New York: Monthly Review Press, 1978.

Ehrenreich, B., and Ehrenreich, J. The new left and the professional-managerial class. In R. Wilson, comp., *Professionals as workers.* Cambridge, Mass.: Policy Training Center, n.d.

Ehrenreich, B., and English, D. *Witches, midwives, and nurses: A history of women healers.* Old Westbury, N.Y.: Feminist Press, 1973.

_____. *For her own good: 150 years of the expert's advice to women.* Garden City, N.Y.: Anchor Press/Doubleday, 1978.

Engel, G. V., and Hall, R. H. The growing industrialization of the professions. In E. Freidson, ed., *The professions and their prospects.* Beverly Hills, Calif.: Sage Publications, 1973.

Erdmann, J. Considerations in extending the validity of the certification process. *Conference on extending the validity of certification.* Chicago: American Board of Medical Specialties, 1976.

Falk, D. S.; Weisfeld, N.; and Tochen, D. *Perspectives on health occupation credentialing: A report of the National Commission for Health Certifying Agencies.* Washington, D.C.: U.S. Government Printing Office, 1980.

Fauri, D. P. The limits on consumer participation in public service programs. In H. Rosen, J. M. Mitsch, and S. Levey, eds., *The consumer in the health care system: Social and managerial perspectives.* New York: Plenum, 1977.

Federal file. *Professional Regulation News.* 1982, *2*(4-5), 1-2.

Federal Trade Commission. *Consumer information remedies: Policy review session.* Washington, D.C.: U.S. Government Printing Office, 1979.

Fine, M. W. The health care system in society. In U.S. Department of Health, Education, and Welfare, *Certification in allied health systems.* Washington, D.C.: U.S. Government Printing Office, 1971.

Frech, H. E. Occupational licensure and health care productivity: The issues and the literature. In J. Rafferty, ed., *Health, manpower, and productivity.* Lexington, Mass.: Lexington Books, 1974.

Freidson, E. *Professional dominance.* New York: Aldine, 1970.

_____, ed. *The professions and their prospects.* Beverly Hills, Calif.: Sage Publications, 1973.

Friedman, M. *Capitalism and freedom.* Chicago: University of Chicago Press, 1962.

Friedman, M., and Friedman, R. *Free to choose.* New York: Harcourt, Brace and Jovanovich, 1980.

Gartner, A., and Riessman, F. *Self-help in the human services.* San Francisco: Jossey-Bass, 1977.

Gellhorn, W. Occupational licensing—A nationwide dilemma. *The Journal of Accountancy,* 1960, *109*(1), 39-45.

_____. The abuse of occupational licensing. *The University of Chicago Law Review,* 1976, *44*(1), 6-27.

Gerstl, J., and Jacobs, G. *Professions for the people.* Cambridge, Mass.: Schenkman, 1976.

Gilb, C. L. *Hidden hierarchies: The professions and government.* New York: Harper & Row, 1966.

Gill, S. J. Professional disclosure and consumer protection in counseling. *Personnel and Guidance Journal,* 1982, *60*(7), 443-46.

Goldfarb v. *Virginia State Bar,* 421 U.S. 733 (1975).

Goldsmith, J. Competence assessment within a professional training program. In P. S. Pottinger and J. Goldsmith, eds., *Defining and measuring competence.* San Francisco: Jossey-Bass, 1979.

Goode, W. J. Encroachment, charlatanism, and the emerging profession: Psychology, sociology, and medicine. *American Sociological Review,* 1960, *25,* 902-14.

Gordon, R. S. *Issues in health care regulation.* New York: McGraw-Hill, 1980.

Grad, F. P., and Marti, N. *Physician's licensure and discipline: The legal and professional regulation of medical practice.* Dobbs Ferry, N.Y.: Oceana Publications, 1979.

Graubard, S. R. Preface to the issue, Doing better and feeling worse: Health in the United States. *Daedalus,* 1977, *106*(1), v-vi.

Green, J. A. Legal issues in a health revolution. In Berkeley Holistic Health Center, *The holistic health handbook.* Berkeley, Calif.: And/Or Press, 1978.

Green, J. A. (with Steven Markell). The health care contract: A model for sharing responsibility. *Somatics,* 1982, *7*(1), 6-15.

Greene, K. Occupational licensing: Protection for whom? *Manpower,* 1969, *1*(6), 2-6.

Greer, S.; Hedlund, R. D.; and Gibson, J. L., eds. *Accountability in urban society.* Beverly Hills, Calif.: Sage Publications, 1978.

Griggs v. *Duke Power Company,* 401 U.S. 424 (1971).

Gross, S. J. Professional disclosure: An alternative to licensing. *Personnel and Guidance Journal,* 1977, *55*(10), 586-88.

Haberfield, S.; Saxby, D.; and Schletter, D. The problem of occupational licensing in perspective. In Department of Consumer Affairs, *Professional licensing in California.* Author, 1978.

Haley, J. Why a mental health clinic should avoid family therapy. *Journal of Marriage and Family Counseling,* 1975, *1,* 3-13.

Hamilton, P. A. *Health care consumerism.* St. Louis: C. V. Mosby, 1982.

Hardcastle, D. A. Public regulation of social work. *Social Work,* 1977, *22,* 14-19.

Harris, R. G. A critical review of "An economic analysis of the regulatory impact of selected boards, bureaus, and commissions." Submitted to the Regulatory Task Force, Department of Consumer Affairs, State of California, March 16, 1978.

Hartley, D.; Roback, H. B.; and Abramowitz, S. I. Deterioration effects in encounter groups. *American Psychologist,* 1976, *31,* 247-55.

Haskell, T. L. *The emergence of professional social science.* Urbana: University of Illinois Press, 1977.

Haug, M., and Sussman, M. Professional autonomy and the revolt of the client. *Social Problems,* 1969, *17*(2), 153-61.

Havighurst, C. C. Anti-trust enforcement in the medical services industry: What does it all mean? *Milbank Memorial Fund Quarterly: Health and Society,* 1980, *58,* 89-124.

_____. *Deregulating the health care industry: Planning for competition.* Cambridge, Mass.: Ballinger, 1982.

Healey, K. The effect of licensure on clinical laboratory effectiveness. Doctoral dissertation, University of California, Los Angeles, 1973. *Dissertation Abstracts International,* 1973, *34,* 2728B.

Heaton, H. *Productivity in service organizations.* New York: McGraw-Hill, 1977.

Henry, W. E.; Sims, J. H.; and Spray, S. L. *The fifth profession.* San Francisco: Jossey-Bass, 1971.

Hogan, D. B. Competence as a facilitator of personal growth groups. *Journal of Humanistic Psychology,* 1977, *17*(2), 33-54.

_____. *The regulation of psychotherapists, Volume I: A study in the philosophy and practice of professional regulation.* Cambridge, Mass.: Ballinger, 1979a.

_____. *The regulation of psychotherapists, Volume II: A handbook of state licensure laws.* Cambridge, Mass.: Ballinger, 1979b.

Holen, A. S. Effects of professional licensing arrangements on interstate labor mobility and resource allocation. *The Journal of Political Economy,* 1965, *73*(5), 492-98.

_____. *The economics of dental licensing.* Arlington, Va.: Public Research Institute of the Center for Naval Analysis, 1978.

Hopewell, L. The system is at fault. *The Public Member* (National Center for the Study of Professions), 1980, 4ff.

Houle, C. O. *Continuing learning in the professions.* San Francisco: Jossey-Bass, 1980.

Hughes, E. C. Professions. In K. S. Lynn, ed., *The professions in America.* Boston: Houghton-Mifflin, 1965.

Illich, I. *Medical nemesis.* New York: Random House, 1976.

Ingle, J. I. Foreword. In P. Milgrom, *Regulation and the quality of dental care.* Germantown, Md.: Aspen Systems Corporation, 1978.

Inglis, B. *The case for unorthodox medicine.* New York: G. P. Putnam & Sons, 1964.

Investigating professionalism. *APA Monitor,* September/October 1978, 8.

Joy, L. Testimony. In N. Ayadi, comp. and ed., Report of the Special Committee to Investigate the Department of Licensing and Regulation. Lansing, Michigan, House of Representatives, 1977.

Kane, M. T. The validity of licensure examinations. *American Psychologist*, 1982, *37*(8), 911-18.

Kessell, R. A. The A.M.A. and the supply of physicians. *Law and Contemporary Problems*, 1970, *35*(2), 267-83.

Kett, J. F. *The formation of the American medical profession: The role of the institutions, 1780-1860*. New Haven, Conn.: Yale University Press, 1968.

Klemp, G. O., Jr. Identifying, measuring, and integrating competence. In P. S. Pottinger and J. Goldsmith, eds., *Defining and measuring competence*. San Francisco: Jossey-Bass, 1979.

Knowles, J. H. Introduction, Doing better and feeling worse. *Daedalus*, 1977, *106*(1), 1-7.

Knox, A. B. Conclusions about impact evaluation. In A. B. Knox, ed., *Assessing the impact of continuing education*. San Francisco: Jossey-Bass, 1979.

Koocher, G. P. Credentialing in psychology: Close encounters with competence. *American Psychologist*, 1979, *34*, 696-702.

Krause, E. A. *Power and illness*. New York: Elsevier, 1977.

La Duca, A. The structure of competence in health professions. *Evaluation and the Health Professions*, 1980, *3*(3), 253-85.

Larson, M. S. *The rise of professionalism: A sociological analysis*. Berkeley: University of California Press, 1977.

Leffler, K. B. Physician licensure: Competition and monopoly in American medicine. *Journal of Law and Economics*, 1978, *21*(1), 165-86.

Legislation regulating professions. *The Journal of Accountancy*, 1960, *109*(1), 27-28.

Lenrow, P. Dilemmas of professional helping: Continuities and discontinuities with folk helping roles. In L. Wispe, ed., *Altruism, sympathy and helping*. New York: Academic Press, 1978.

Levin, L. S.; Katz, A. H.; and Holst, E. *Self-care: Lay initiative in health*. 2d ed. New York: Prodist, 1979.

Levin, T. *American health: Professional privilege vs. public need*. New York: Praeger, 1974.

Licensure efforts of dubious benefit to health groups. *Professional Regulation News*, 1982, *2*(4-5), 10-11.

Lieberman, J. K. *The tyranny of the experts*. New York: Walker & Co., 1970.

Lindenberg, S. P. Attention students. Be advised. . . . *Personnel and Guidance Journal*, 1976, *55*, 34-36.

Lipsky, M. The assault on human services: Street level bureaucrats accountability, and the fiscal crisis. In S. Greer, R. D. Hedlund, and J. L. Gibson, eds., *Accountability in urban society*. Beverly Hills, Calif.: Sage Publications, 1978.

Litoff, J. B. *American midwives: 1860 to the present*. Westport, Conn.: Greenwood Press, 1978.

Lopata, H. Z. Expertization of everyone and the revolt of the client. *The Sociological Quarterly*, 1976, *17*(4), 435-47.

McClelland, D. C. Testing for competence rather than "intelligence." *American Psychologist*, 1973, *28*(1), 1-14.

McClelland, D. C., and Boyatzis, R. E. Opportunities for counselors from the competency assessment movement. *Personnel and Guidance Journal*, 1980, *58*(5), 368-72.

McGaghie, W. C. The evaluation of competence. *Evaluation and the Health Professions*, 1980, *3*(3), 289-320.

McGuire, C. H. A process approach to the construction and analysis of medical examinations. *Journal of Medical Education*, 1963, *38*(7), 556-63.

———. A scientific approach to problems of professional assessment. *Canadian Medical Association Journal*, 1969, *100*(13), 593-98.

Mackin, P. K. Occupational licensing: A warning. *Personnel and Guidance Journal*, 1976, *54*, 507ff.

McKinlay, J., and Dutton, D. B. Social-psychological factors affecting health service utilization. In S. J. Mushkin, ed., *Consumer incentives for health care*. New York: Prodist, 1974.

McLaughlin v. Florida, 379 U.S. 184 (1964).

Magaro, P. A.; Gripp, R.; McDowell, D. J.; and Miller, I. W. III. *The mental health industry: A cultural phenomenon*. New York: Wiley, 1978.

Makofsky, D. Malpractice and medicine. *Society*, 1977, *14*(2), 25-29.

Marieskind, H. I. Helping oneself to health. *Social Policy*, 1976, *7*(2), 63-66.

———. *Women in the health system: Patients, providers, and programs*. St. Louis: Mosby, 1980.

Martin, D. L. Will the sun set on occupational licensing? In S. Rottenberg, ed., *Occupational licensure and regulation*. Washington, D.C.: American Enterprise Institute, 1980.

Maurizi, A. Occupational licensure and the public interest. *Journal of Political Economy*, 1974, *82*, 399-413.

———. *Quality impacts: Complaints to regulatory boards. An economic analysis of the regulatory impact of selected boards, bureaus, and commissions.* A report to the Office of the Director of the California Department of Consumer Affairs, 1977a, 30-65.

———. *Quality impacts: Complaints to the Structural Pest Board. An economic analysis of the regulatory impact of selected boards, bureaus, and commissions.* A report to the Office of the Director of the California Department of Consumer Affairs, 1977b, 66-130.

———. *Quality impacts: Complaints to the Contractor's Board. An economic analysis of the regulatory impact of selected boards, bureaus, and commissions.* A report to the Office of the Director of the California Department of Consumer Affairs, 1977c, 131-57.

———. The impact of regulations on quality: The case of the California contractors. In S. Rottenberg, ed., *Occupational licensure and regulation*. Washington, D.C.: American Enterprise Institute, 1980.

Mechanic, D. *The growth of bureaucratic medicine*. New York: Wiley, 1976.

———. *Future issues in health care*. New York: Free Press, 1979.

Menne, J. W. Competency based assessment and the profession of psychology. *Professional Practice of Psychology*, 1981, *2*(1), 17-22.

Messick, S. Test validity and the ethics of assessment. *American Psychologist*, 1980, *35*(11), 1012-27.

Milgrom, P. *Regulation and the quality of dental care*. Germantown, Md.: Aspen Systems Corporation, 1978.

Moore, T. G. The purpose of licensing. *Journal of Law and Economics*, 1961, *4*, 93-117.

Moore, W. S. Introduction, Part two, Sunset review. In T. B. Clark et al., eds., *Reforming regulation*. Washington, D.C.: American Enterprise Institute, 1980.

Morrison, J. K. A consumer-oriented approach to psychotherapy. *Psychotherapy: Theory, Research, and Practice*, 1979, *16*, 381-84.

Muris, T. J., and McChesney, F. S. Advertising and the price and quality of legal services: The case of legal claims. *American Bar Association Research Journal*, 1979, 179-207.

National Academies of Practice formed. *Professional Regulation News*, 1982, *1*(10), 2-3.

National Advisory Commission on Health Manpower. *Report, Volume II*. Washington, D.C.: U.S. Government Printing Office, 1967.

Newman, S. A., and Kramer, N. *Getting what you deserve*. Garden City, N.Y.: Doubleday, 1979.

Ng, L.K.I.; Davis, D. L.; and Manderscheid, R. W. The Health Promotion Organization: A practical intervention designed to promote healthy living. *Public Health Reports*, 1978, *93*(5), 446-55.

Office of Technology Assessment. *Assessing the efficacy and safety of medical technologies*. Washington, D.C.: U.S. Government Printing Office, 1978.

On the dental front. *ProForum*, 1979, *1*(12), 5.

Overcast, T. D.; Sales, B. D.; and Pollard, M. R. Applying anti-trust laws to the professions: Implications for psychology. *American Psychologist*, 1982, *37*(5), 517-25.

Parloff, M. B. Can psychotherapy research guide the policymaker? *American Psychologist*, 1979, *34*(4), 296-306.

Pashigian, B. P. Has occupational licensing reduced geographical mobility and raised earnings? In S. Rottenberg, ed., *Occupational licensure and regulation*. Washington, D.C.: American Enterprise Institute, 1980.

Passarelli, A. Credentialing in nursing: Background issues. In American Nurses Association, *The study of credentialing in nursing: A new approach, Volume II. Staff working paper*. Kansas City: Association, 1979.

Paxton, A. Self-help: Professional crisis or challenge? *ProForum*, 1979, *1*(12), 1ff.

_____. Taking license: Where continuing competence matters. *ProForum*, 1982, *4*(4), 12ff.

Payne, P. E. Licensure: Professions and occupations. Report to the Commerce Committee, House of Representatives, State of Washington, Olympia, 1977.

Pennell, M. Y. and Hoover, D. B. Health manpower source book 21: Allied health manpower supply and requirements: 1950-1980. Washington, D.C.: U.S. Government Printing Office, 1970.

Pennell, M. Y., and Stewart, P. A. *State licensing of health occupations*. Public Health Service publication #1758. Washington, D.C.: U.S. Government Printing Office, 1968.

Pertschuk, M. Needs and licenses. In S. Rottenberg, ed., *Occupational licensure and regulation*. Washington, D.C.: American Enterprise Institute, 1980.

Peter, L. J. *Peter's quotations: Ideas for our time*. New York: William Morrow, 1977.

Pfeffer, J. Some evidence on occupational licensing and occupational incomes. *Social Forces*, 1974, *53*, 102-11.

Phelan, J. J. *Economic report on the regulation of the television repair industry in Louisiana and California*. Washington, D.C.: U.S. Government Printing Office, 1974.

Pottinger, P. S. Competence testing as a basis for licensing: Problems and prospects. Paper presented at the Conference on Credentialism, University of California Law School, Berkeley, California, April 1977.

_____. An issue has come of age. *ProForum*, 1979a, *1*(10), 8ff.

_____. Truth in testing: How will the professions score? *ProForum*, 1979b, *2*(3)), 8.

_____. Competence assessment: Comments on current practices. In P. S. Pottinger and J. Goldsmith, eds., *Defining and measuring competence.* San Francisco: Jossey-Bass, 1979c.

_____. Laying down the law. *ProForum*, 1980a, *2*(12), 3.

_____. Proficiency testing: A study in disharmony. *ProForum*, 1980b, *2*(10), 14.

Priestley, P.; McGuire, J.; Flagg, D.; Hemsley, V.; and Welham, D. *Social skills and personal problem solving.* London: Tavistock Publications, 1978.

Proposal for revision of Section 2052 of the Medical Practice Act. Sacramento, Calif.: Board of Medical Quality Assurance, 1982.

Rappaport, J. Education, training, and dealing with the contingent future. Presentation at a meeting of the American Psychological Association, Toronto, 1978.

Reiff, R. The control of knowledge: The power of the helping professions. *Journal of Applied Behavioral Science,* 1974, *10*(3), 451-61.

Riessman, F. "Consumerizing" health care. *ProForum*, 1979, *2*, 8ff.

Roederer, D., and Palmer, B. *Sunset: Expectation and experience.* Lexington, Ky.: Council of State Governments, 1981.

Roederer, D., and Shimberg, B. *Occupational licensing: Centralizing state licensure functions.* Lexington, Ky.: Council of State Governments, 1980.

Roemer, M. Controling and promoting quality in medical care. *Law and Contemporary Problems,* 1970, *35*(2), 284-304.

Roemer, R. Legal systems regulating health personnel. In J. B. McKinlay, ed., *Politics and law in health policy.* New York: Prodist, 1973.

_____. Trends in licensure, certification, and accreditation: Implications for health manpower education in the future. *Journal of Applied Health,* 1974, *3,* 26-33.

Rogers, C. R. Some new challenges. *American Psychologist,* 1973, *28,* 379-87.

Rosen, H.; Metsch, J.; and Levy, S. *The consumer and the health care system: Social and managerial perspectives.* New York: Spectrum Publications, 1977.

Rosner, J. F. Self-regulation in the dental profession. *Journal of the American Dental Association,* 1979, *98*(6), 919-24.

Roth, J. A. Recruitment, training, and certification in emerging health role. Paper presented at the American Association for the Advancement of Science, New York, January 31, 1975.

Sarason, S. B., and Lorentz, E. *The challenge of the resource exchange network.* San Francisco: Jossey-Bass, 1979.

Schenkel, K. F. *Report on the conference of professional assessment.* American Psychological Association Board of Professional Affairs, Washington, D.C.: February 1980.

Shepard, L. Licensing restrictions and the cost of dental care. *Journal of Law and Economics,* 1978, *21*(1), 187-201.

Shimberg, B. The sunset approach: The key to regulatory reform. *State Government,* 1976, *49,* 140-47.

_____. Continuing education and licensing. In D. W. Vermilye, ed., *Relating work and education.* San Francisco: Jossey-Bass, 1977.

_____. *Recruiting and selecting members for occupational licensing boards*. Remarks before advisory committee appointed by Governor Graham to recommend individuals for board membership, Tallahassee, Fla.: April 11, 1979.

_____. *National developments in health occupations credentialing*. Statewide Health Occupations Education Review Committee, Institute for Research and Development in Occupational Education, Graduate School and University Center, City University of New York, Buffalo: December 1980.

_____. Testing for licensure and certification. *American Psychologist*, 1981, *36*(10), 1138-44.

_____. *Occupational licensing: A public perspective*. Princeton, N.J.: Educational Testing Service, 1982.

_____. What is competence? How can it be assessed? In M. R. Stern, ed., *Power and conflict in continuing professional education*. Belmont, Calif.: Wadsworth, 1983.

Shimberg, B.; Esser, B. F.; and Krueger, D. H. *Occupational licensing*. Washington, D.C.: Public Affairs Press, 1973.

Shryock, R. H. *Medical licensing in America, 1650-1965*. Baltimore: Johns Hopkins Press, 1967.

Smith, M. L., and Glass, G. V. Meta-analysis of psychotherapy outcome studies. *American Psychologist*, 1977, *32*, 752-60.

Somers, A. R. Comment. In W. Greenburg, ed., *Competition in the health care sector: Past, present, and future*. Proceedings of a conference sponsored by the Bureau of Economics, Federal Trade Commission: March 1978.

Somers, A. R., and Somers, H. M. *Health and health care*. Germantown, Md.: Aspen Systems Corporation, 1977.

Sorkin, A. L. *Health manpower: An economic perspective*. Lexington, Mass.: Lexington Books, 1977.

Special projects report. . . . Psychology comes of age. *Advance*, 1979, August-September, 7.

Spiegel, A. D., and Backhaut, B. H. *Curing and caring: A review of the factors affecting the quality and acceptability of health care*. New York: Spectrum, 1980.

Stephens, M. *The status of sunset in the states: A Common Cause report*. Washington, D.C.: Common Cause, 1982.

Stevens, J. The coming physician surplus. *Journal of the American Dietetic Association*, 1982, *80*(3), 245-47.

Stewart, P. L., and Cantor, M. G. *Varieties of work experience*. New York: John Wiley & Sons, 1974.

Stigler, G. J. The theory of economic regulation. *The Bell Journal of Economics and Management Science*, 1971, *2*(1), 3-21.

The study of credentialing in Virginia: A new approach: Volume II, staff working papers. Kansas City: American Nurses Association, 1979.

Sugarman v. Dugall, 413 U.S. 634 (1973).

Summerfield, H. L. *Review of Psychology Examining Committee and State Board of Behavioral Science Examiners: A report of the Regulatory Review Task Force*. State of California, Department of Consumer Affairs: 1978.

Swain, K. L. Marriage and family counselor licensure: Special reference to Nevada. *Journal of Marriage and Family Counseling*, 1975, *1*, 149-55.

Swanson, C. D. A case supporting licensure. *APGA Guidepost*, August 19, 1976, 5.

Swanson, J. L. Counseling Directory and Consumer's Guide: Implementing professional disclosure and consumer protection. *Personnel and Guidance Journal*, 1979, *58*(3), 190-93.

Sweeney, T. J., and Sturdevant, A. D. Licensure in the helping professions: Anatomy of an issue. *Personnel and Guidance Journal*, 1974, *52*(9), 575-80.

Szasz, T. *The theology of medicine*. Baton Rouge: Louisiana State University Press, 1977.

Tabachnik, L. Licensing in the legal and medical professions, 1820-1860: A historical case study. In J. Gerstl and G. Jacobs, eds., *Professions for the people*. New York: Schenkman, 1976.

Tennov, D. *Psychotherapy: The hazardous cure*. New York: Abelard-Schuman, 1975.

Theobold, R. *Habit and habitat*. Englewood Cliffs, N.J.: Prentice-Hall, 1972.

Tochen, D. K. *Occupational licensing: A new role for consumers*. Washington, D.C.: Paul H. Douglas Consumer Research Center, 1978.

Ullman, D. Regulate freedom of choice: An alternative to scope of practice licensure. Paper presented at the American Public Health Association Conference, Detroit, November 1981.

Virginia licensing study criticizes complaint handling, "questionable standards." *Professional Regulation News*, 1982, *2*(3), 4-5.

Waddle, F. Licensure: Achievements and limitations. In *The study of credentialing in nursing: A new approach. Volume II, staff working papers*. Kansas City: American Nurses Association, 1979.

Welch, C. E. Quality care, quasi-care, and quackery. *Proceedings of the Institute of Medicine of Chicago*, 1973, *29*, 412-18.

White, W. D. *Public health and private gain: The economics of licensing clinical laboratory personnel*. Chicago: Maaroufa Press, 1979a.

_____. Why is regulation introduced in the health sector? Look at occupational licensure. *Journal of Health Politics, Policy and Law*, 1979b, *3*, 536-52.

Whitesel, R. *Regulation and licensing: An overview*. Legislative Council Staff Research Bulletin 76-7. Madison, Wisc.: 1977.

Williamson, J. W. Validation by performance measures. In American Board of Medical Specialities, *Conference on extending the validity of certification*. Chicago: Board, 1976.

Wilson, J. Q. *The politics of regulation*. New York: Basic Books, 1980.

Winborn, B. B. Honest labelling and other procedures for the protection of consumers of counseling. *Personnel and Guidance Journal*, 1977, *56*(4), 206-9.

INDEX

About the Author

STANLEY J. GROSS is Professor of Counseling Psychology at Indiana State University. He has contributed articles on professional licensing to *Power and Conflict in Continuing Education, Journal of Holistic Medicine, American Psychologist,* and *Personnel and Guidance Journal.*